The Morning After

Teens Write About Sex and Unplanned Pregnancy

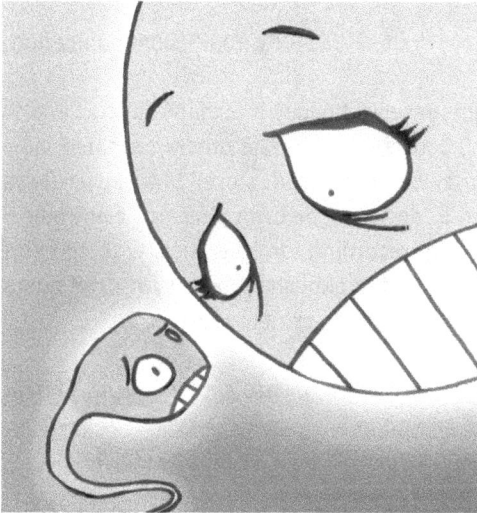

By Youth Communication

Edited by Maria Luisa Tucker

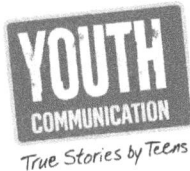

YOUTH COMMUNICATION

True Stories by Teens

The Morning After

EXECUTIVE EDITORS
Keith Hefner and Laura Longhine

CONTRIBUTING EDITORS
Kendra Hurley, Clarence Haynes, Rachel Blustain, Andrea Estepa,
Philip Kay, and Nora McCarthy

LAYOUT & DESIGN
Efrain Reyes, Jr. and Jeff Faerber

COVER ART
Karolina Zaniesienko

ISBN 978-1-935552-36-9

Second, Expanded Edition

Printed in the United States of America

Youth Communication ®
New York, New York
www.youthcomm.org

Catalog Item #YD28-1

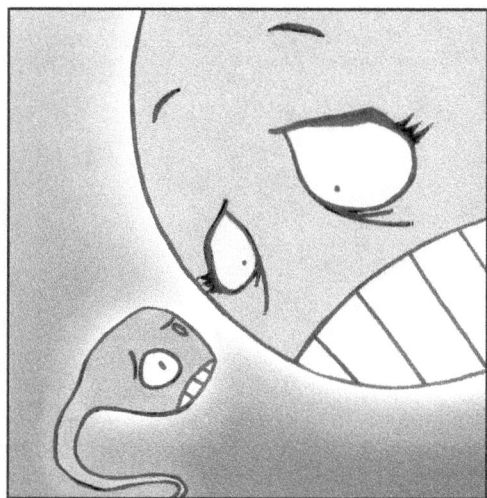

Table of Contents

A Difficult Decision

> *Facing an unplanned pregnancy at 16, the writer realizes she's not ready to be a mother and opts for an abortion.*

Keeping My Baby

> *The writer gets pregnant at 16 and decides to have the baby. She's wants a child to love, but she's also worried about becoming a mother.*

A Choice I Couldn't Make

> *Only 14, DeAnna doesn't know what to do when she finds out she's pregnant. She's both angry and relieved when her mother makes the decision for her.*

Why I Always Use a Condom

> *The writer has unprotected sex with his girlfriend. She becomes pregnant, has the baby, and cuts off all contact with the writer, who is devastated by guilt and anger.*

If You Believe These Lines, Check the Price of Pampers

> *Frank gives tips on how to respond to common lines teens use to pressure their partners into having unprotected sex.*

Back in the Stirrups—Again

> *Madeleine gives a clear, comprehensive, and reassuring explanation of what happens during a GYN exam.*

All About Birth Control, Right Here

> *Detailed information on the pros and cons of various contraceptives.*

> *The facts on parenting, adoption, and abortion.*

Using the Book

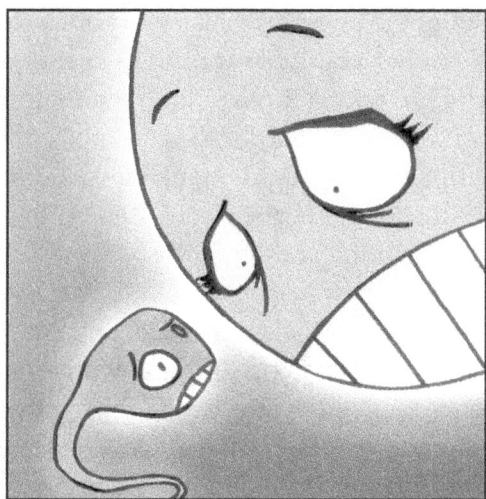

Introduction

One-third of American girls get pregnant at least once by the time they are 20, and the vast majority of those pregnancies are unplanned.* We all know the difficult choices these young women face: ending the pregnancy, teen parenthood, or giving the baby up for adoption. As the true stories here attest, each choice carries its own burden.

In "Growing Up Together," Vanessa Sanchez, pregnant at 18, decides to keep her child. She provides readers with a glimpse into her hectic life with a 3-year-old. "The first few months after John was born were a lot harder than I expected," she writes. She struggles with sleepless nights, loneliness, self-doubt, and how to effectively discipline her son. "I [used to think] 'I'll just talk to him about discipline and he'll follow what I say,'" she writes. "Little did I know it wasn't that easy." The 16-year-old author of "Keeping My Baby" also decides to take on motherhood because, she says, abortion or adoption would haunt her forever. However, she is plagued by anxiety, worrying that she will repeat the same bad patterns of her own abusive parents.

Several other teens write about the decision to have an abortion. The 17-year-old author of "The Right Choice for Me—for Now" is shocked to discover she's pregnant after having protected sex with her ex-boyfriend. Panicked, she tells her mother and ultimately decides to end the pregnancy. "My heart still aches when I think about it," she writes. "I want to have a baby when I meet the right man and it's the right time for me. But it's not that time yet."

Other teens who don't feel prepared for parenthood decide on adoption. In "A Family to Raise Her," Jennifer Jeanne Olensky writes about why this choice felt right for her and her baby, despite how difficult it was. "In giving [my baby] up, I gave two loving people the family they longed for, my daughter a chance to thrive, and myself the opportunity to grow and become the person I am now."

Other stories remind us that mothers aren't the only ones whose lives are altered by unplanned pregnancy. In "Mom Wasn't Ready for Me," the child of a teen mom reflects on how her mother's decision impacted her own life. She writes: "I don't think [my mom] realized how difficult it is to be a mom while you're still trying to grow up yourself. She hopped and skipped right over her childhood, and then she stumbled, and we, her kids, struggled with her."

In "Why I Always Use a Condom," a teen father laments both his carelessness and his distant relationship with his young son. "We should have used a condom that day," the author writes. "Not only to protect ourselves, but to protect everyone around us who was affected by our behavior."

These writers offer a variety of perspectives on teen pregnancy, but the same feeling is echoed in each of their stories: regret.

These tales are not meant to scold teens who decide to have sex, or to promote any particular response to unplanned pregnancy—parenthood, abortion, and adoption are deeply personal choices. Rather, we hope these stories will help teens make conscious decisions about whether or not to have sex, and how to protect themselves, *before* being faced with its consequences.

In the following stories, names have been changed: *Three Tales of Teen Pregnancy, The Morning After, Mom Wasn't Ready for Me, The Right Choice for Me—for Now, Am I the Father?, Stressed About Sex, There's More to Sex Than Sex, A Difficult Decision, Keeping My Baby,* and *Why I Always Use a Condom.*

*According to the National Campaign to Prevent Teen and Unplanned Pregnancy

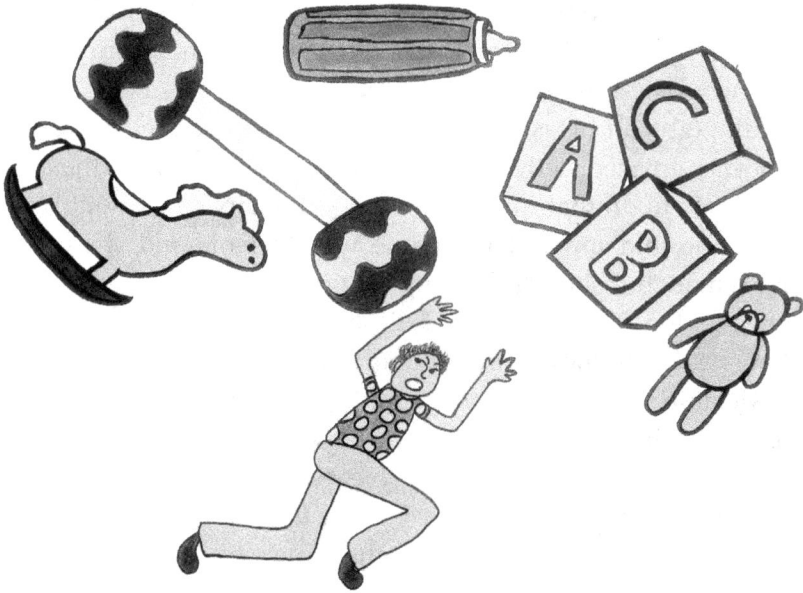

Stephanie "Meadow" Kunar

Am I the Father?

By Anonymous

One day in June, I received a phone call from a female acquaintance. We were conversing normally until she came out of nowhere and said, "I'm pregnant and I think it's yours." My eyes opened wide, and I asked her when this happened. "Remember back on October 2?" she said.

I was stunned as I remembered the night she was talking about. Then I couldn't think too well because anger came over me. I asked loudly, "How long did you know this? How many months are you?"

She told me that the baby was due next week and I was the father. I was furious. I couldn't believe she had known this for nine months and was telling me only a week before the baby was due. I hung up on her.

I sat there trying to get my thoughts together. I knew the

night she was talking about. In October, I was chilling and getting drunk at a party when I saw her across the room. I approached her and asked how she was doing. She said, "I've been eyeing you all night, and was waiting for you to come to me."

I was amazed. I thought, "Oh really? Damn. That means I don't have to do that much." We went upstairs so we could talk alone. She told me that her name was Melanie and she didn't have a man, but she was looking for one. I said I was looking for someone, too. That was a lie. I did have a woman, but I figured what she didn't know wouldn't hurt her.

Melanie started telling me about her life. She said her moms was a pain in the behind. She had an older brother who didn't care too much about her. I was interested in her tale. She said, "Let me get your number and we can talk on the phone sometime." I saw nothing wrong with that. She was cool enough and cute.

Then next thing I knew she started to fall asleep next to me. I tried to wake her up, and she pulled me toward her. We stared into each other's eyes for a hot second, and before I knew it she was kissing my cheek. We were both drunk, and we did our thang.

I felt weird after we had sex. I hadn't had a one-night stand before. I felt like I straight up took advantage of her, and that seemed strange. After we were done, I left her and we never spoke again. Whenever I heard about her through mutual friends, I just thought of her as a female I met at a party.

But now she had called me, nine months later, to tell me a baby had come out of that night and that it would be in the world in a week. I was confused. I wanted to punch something.

Instead, I called my new girl, who I had only recently started seeing, and told her what was going down. My lady sounded stunned on the phone but helped me think through the situation. We both thought that the first thing I needed to do was to take a paternity test to see if the kid was really mine. We weren't ready yet to think too far beyond that. I kept asking myself, "What if it is mine? Am I ready to be a father? Am I ready to take care of another life?"

I did know that if it was mine, I wasn't going to abandon it. I've seen too many fathers leave their kids behind. In fact, my own father left me behind when he went to jail. I knew the pain of growing up without a dad, and I always swore I wouldn't do that if I had a child. But I knew if I became a father, my teenage life was gone. I would have to stop acting like a boy and take care of my responsibilities as a man.

I didn't know what that meant, exactly. I didn't know whether it meant I would have to quit school to get a full-time job. I did know I was too young for this. What's worse, I didn't have a penny to my name. But the baby would need things: diapers, a crib, toys, clothes, milk.

I had some idea about how hard it is to be a good parent. After all, neither of my parents pulled it off well enough to keep me at home.

There were so many thoughts in my head, so many things to do, and I didn't have much time to do those things. The walls were closing in quickly and I felt I had no one to help me. I couldn't go back to selling products on the street. What good would I be to my kid if I were dead or locked up? I couldn't go to my parents. They would kill me. How the hell could I tell my moms that I had a kid? How could I tell any of my family members? I was ashamed. I was supposed to be the one who succeeded, who didn't get caught up in situations like this.

The only thing I knew was that I wanted to be part of this kid's life. No matter what the circumstances were, I wasn't leaving my seed. But how was I ever going to handle getting along with the kid's mother, someone who would be there in the child's life forever, someone I couldn't stand for putting me through this?

Melanie called me back and asked why I hung up on her. I told her, "You knew all this and held out on me for this long, and you're wondering why I'm being mean to you? I want nothing to do with you. I want to be with my lady and that's it. The only reason I am going be nice to you and show some respect toward you is for the kid."

I knew I was half responsible for all this, and that made me even angrier.

At the time graduation was coming up, and I had to pass the tests I needed to graduate. As I was studying for the tests and, later, taking them, my mind was on the baby. I could think of nothing but the baby, my girl, my family, and how was I going to make money.

For a while I thought that my girl would leave me to avoid dealing with baby mama drama. "Why would I leave?" she said when I told her what I was afraid of. "I said I was going to be there for you and that's what I'm doing."

My friends who knew about the baby situation were shocked about the news, but they also supported me 100%. I couldn't ask for better friends in a time of need. But that didn't mean everything was good. I was nervous just thinking about becoming a father, and even with the best friends and girl in the world, I wasn't ready.

It's frightening to look at something so small and know how much it needs you.

I had some idea about how hard it is to be a good parent. After all, neither of my parents pulled it off well enough to keep me at home, and I ended up in foster care. It hurt that my father had always been in and out of my life.

Previously, when I'd thought of having kids myself, I imagined that everything would be perfect. I wanted to have two, a boy and a girl, or as I would call them, my prince and princess. I pictured having my kids by the wife I chose to marry, and being financially stable enough to take care of them. I didn't want things to be like this—to have a baby by someone who I didn't care for, and to raise a kid when I'm not stable.

On Thursday, June 20, Melanie had the baby. She called me two hours after she delivered and told me that it was a boy. I was happy to hear that it had gone well with her and that the baby was healthy.

I went to the hospital that Friday to take the paternity test. As he took some blood for my DNA, the doctor said the results wouldn't be ready for a few days. I felt weird having the blood drawn; my arm was flinching as he did it. I couldn't stop thinking about how all of this was happening so fast.

Afterward, I went to see the baby. He was sleeping and beautiful. The last time I saw a baby that beautiful was when my little sister was born. I asked the nurse if I could hold him, and she gave me the baby. I sat there holding Shorty in my arms like a prized possession. I started talking to the baby like I already knew he was mine. He was cute, with hazel eyes, a little hair, and tiny hands and feet.

When the nurse told me that she had to put him back in the crib, I didn't want to let him go. The whole feeling that the baby was mine hit me hard. I saw Shorty's eyes and I knew that I would be ready for this. He was my responsibility and I wouldn't let him down.

The whole time I was in the hospital room, Melanie and I didn't communicate. The only time we spoke was when it regarded the baby. I told Melanie, "My only plans are to raise that baby, nothing else." She said she understood that. I told her I would get the diapers and some toys, though I still hadn't figured out how.

She said I could see the kid whenever I wanted. I said I'd see Shorty after school and some nights that I had free. Melanie's mom was in the hospital, too. She seemed to like me, but she was also mad at me because she knew that we were too young and that we weren't ready for this.

The Morning After

Monday was the big day, the day I'd find out if the kid was really mine. At the end of the day, I was supposed to meet my lady and tell her the results. When I got to the hospital, I saw Shorty moving, and I asked the doctor if I could hold him while he went and got the results. So I sat there in a chair holding Shorty in my arms, rocking back and forth.

I started talking to him, telling him, "Hey, little one, I might be your father," and, "Don't worry, I will never leave you." I knew I was getting a little too mushy with Shorty, but I couldn't help it. I even felt the urge to cry and let some feelings out. The way the baby moved in my arms was a joyous feeling to me. He was lying there sleeping, eyes closed, his little fists tight. I couldn't believe this was mine.

After a while, Melanie caught my attention. She was just outside the room, and I saw that she was crying. Her mother got up and started yelling at the doctor, "It has to be him." I walked toward them, and as the yelling got louder, the baby started crying and the nurse took him away. Melanie's mother told the doctor, "I'll pay you to tell him he is the father." I couldn't believe what I was hearing. Then I felt like I was about to flip out on her.

As I struggled to stay calm, the doctor pulled me to the side and told me eye to eye, face to face, that the child wasn't mine. I felt strange—both sad and overjoyed. I knew I wasn't ready to be a father, but I had started to like the idea of having a kid to call mine.

That night, I told my girl the news. She was glad. But later as I walked down the streets, I noticed all the babies who were with their fathers, and I started to miss Shorty. It was hard to believe, all I'd been through in the last week because of that one-night mistake with Melanie. It was weird to think that I could've been a father.

I call Melanie once in a while to check up on Shorty. I was mad at her for doing all that to me, but I came out all right while she is giving up her teen years. To be honest, I believe some good has come out of it for me. My lady and I are stronger as a couple after going through that together, and I'm much more cautious about sex. I always use a condom. I know that having kids isn't my thing, not now. (Maybe when I am about 22 and financially stable, I'll think about it.)

After seeing Shorty and holding him in my arms, I see the love fathers have for their kids. But I also see why so many run. It's frightening to look at something so small and know how much it needs you. But that don't make it right for fathers to leave.

The author was in high school when he wrote this story.
He later graduated and went to college.

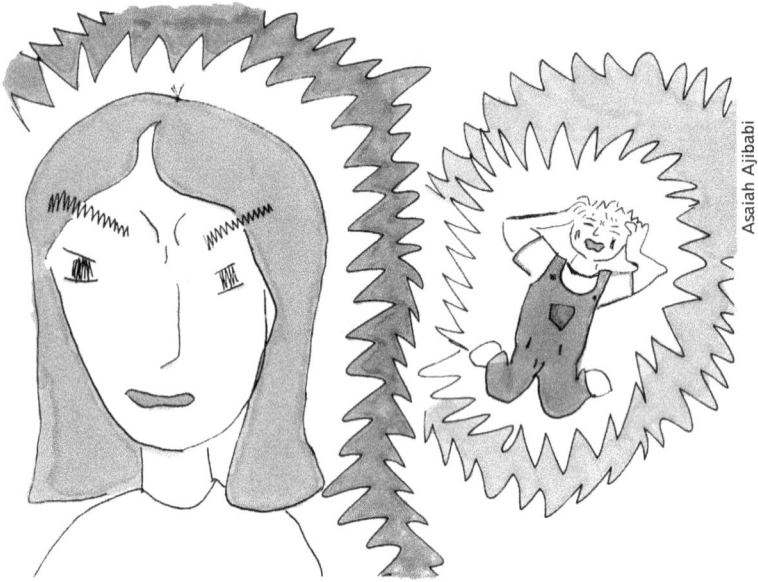

Asaiah Ajibabi

Growing Up Together

By Vanessa Sanchez

One day I went to the supermarket with my 3-year-old son, John, and he started screaming at the top of his lungs. I tried to remain calm.

"John, do you really think that's necessary?" I asked. "Do you even know why you're crying?" But that didn't stop him. He cried as if someone was beating him. It felt like we had a huge, bright spotlight on us in the middle of the jam-packed supermarket. My friend, who was shopping with me, slowly but surely drifted away, as if she was not with us. Everything seemed like a blur of embarrassment as my son cried and cried. I didn't know what to do. I moved into an empty aisle and started yelling with a stern voice.

"If you do not be quiet, I will leave you right here on your own!"

Finally, I took a deep breath, hugged my son, and said, "I love you, John. You are embarrassing the both of us, so if there is something you need, you have to say it, because I cannot understand you when you're crying."

"I'm tired, Mommy," John replied.

"It can't be that simple, John," I sighed, but it was. So I removed my coat and made it into a pillow for him in the shopping cart.

Sometimes it is extremely difficult to handle my son's temper along with mine. The good things—that smile he has, the moments when we connect—keep me going.

I was 18 when I found out I was pregnant with my son. I was one of those stupid little teenagers who wanted a baby because I thought it would be cute. I didn't know then how difficult it would be to raise a child on my own. I didn't realize there would be times when I would feel lonelier than I ever had before, with no one to blame but myself because I made the decision to have a baby.

When I got pregnant, I was determined to be a better mother to John than my own mother had been to me. My mom used drugs when I was a child, and my childhood was sad and embarrassing, from the beatings she gave me to the jokes at school for wearing Payless shoes. My mother was so caught up in her drug habit that our Christmas gifts were given to us and sold in the same day.

Sometimes I catch myself doing the same things awful things my mother did.

I wanted prove to myself and other people that growing up in a negative environment doesn't mean you can't flourish. I plan to raise my son without abusing him in any way, finish college, and pursue a career as a nurse.

To prepare to be a mother, I participated in parenting classes and read books about parenting. One day, I saw a woman on the bus slap her son's hand because he was jumping on the seats. "That's not how I am going to be with my child," I told myself. "I'll just talk to him about discipline and he'll follow what I say."

Yeah, right. Little did I know it wasn't that easy.

The first few months after John was born were a lot harder than I expected. With a newborn, you're lucky if you get a full three hours of sleep. One day John just started crying and crying. I had no idea what was wrong. I mean, I burped, changed, fed, and rocked him, but nothing helped.

Finally, I had no choice but to put him down and walk away because I was literally shaking and dizzy. It took a while before I pulled myself together and said, "If I don't do it, no one else will." I got up, grabbed my baby, and paced for about an hour more until he stopped crying.

The first few months after John was born were a lot harder than I expected.

About two months after John was born, I was finally catching some ZZZs, but things were not going exactly according to plan. By the time John was 2, I was already behind in college. Taking care of my baby, working, and going to school turned out to be nearly impossible. I had to put school off.

Now John is 3 years old. He has a big head topped off with a mat of brown hair, big brown eyes, and two handfuls of cheeks. His little voice brings me an array of feelings, from joy to frustration. I love my son but, boy, does he do some things. He is tougher to discipline now that he's older. I say, "John, don't do that." He says, "You don't do that!"

I get repeated complaints from the teacher: "Your son is being disruptive" or "John does not focus on his work." One day John's teacher said he hit a little girl and she put him in time out. John was so angry that he kept cutting the teacher off to say, "But mom, Victoria bumped me with her butt against the wall!" I wasn't sure who to believe. I was just upset that my baby kept getting into trouble. I'm afraid of my son learning negative patterns of behavior from me, his father, or our families.

For example, one day I was arguing with John's father while cooking sausages on the stove. When they started to burn I said, "I'm not dealing with that," but he did nothing. Smoke started to fill the kitchen. I got so mad that I flung the pot against the kitchen door. My son was watching cartoons in the next room and walked in to see sausages on the floor and his mommy upset.

"What happened, Ma? You all right?" he asked. I quickly had to grab my composure and say yes. I thought, "He's going to learn that this is how to react to anger." That really bothered me. I felt embarrassed that I'd lost control.

Worse, I sometimes catch myself doing the same awful things my mother did. Because of her addiction, my mom was inconsistent. I often felt frustrated that I couldn't count on her to cook when I was hungry or help me with my homework. She disciplined my siblings and me when it wasn't necessary, and let us get away with things when we needed discipline.

Now, inconsistency is the biggest mistake I make with my son. If John jumps on the bed I punish him, but if I'm on the phone and he jumps on the bed then I completely disregard it. I know consistency is difficult, especially for a single parent, but I feel upset that I'm not on top of things as much as I'd like to be.

What I've learned is that parenting is all about confusion. I'm always confused about little things, like whether I should give John a time out, or whether to give him juice when bedtime is around the corner. Should I say no, or do I say no too often?

I'm also confused about the big things: which school to put him in, whether John is learning the right behavior from me, and whether he's growing into a good kid.

I look for signs that John is doing well. I see that he has good qualities: he's loving, helpful, and entertaining. Our communication has developed so we understand each other better now.

Just the other day I was sick and he came and rubbed my

back, saying, "Mommy, you all right?" I was feeling half dead, but I was able to crack a smile, because my baby came along with a thermometer saying, "Turn over, mommy, I'll help you."

Now I understand why people say, "You're too young!" Being a single mother is something you need to be mentally prepared for. My advice to other girls is to wait.

But I also like that my son is here with me through my own years of growing. I started college again in the fall, and over my winter break I kept John home from pre-school most days. I wanted the extra time with him. I am bored at home with no one to tell "Stop that!" or "Come play ball with me."

There are times when John and I are home and I say to myself, "Wow, my baby is growing so fast." I know I have to keep growing at a fast pace, too, to be the mother I want to be. I'm determined to set us both on the right path and make my son proud. John will be there to see me finish college and will be learning from me as I start a career.

Vanessa wrote this story for Rise, *a magazine by and for parents involved in the foster care system. Copyright © Rise magazine. Reprinted with permission. www.risemagazine.org.*

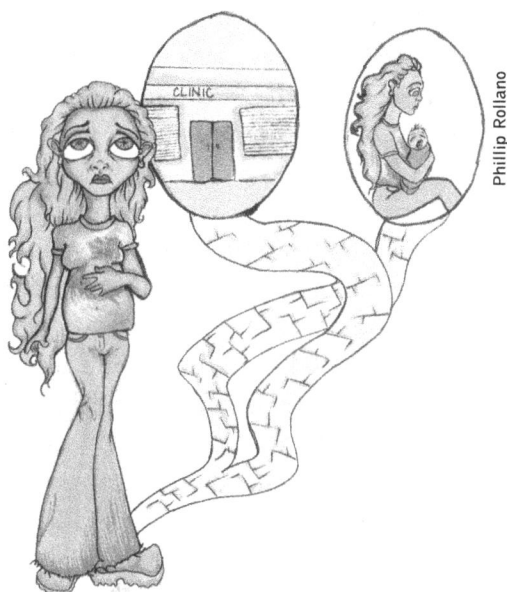

Phillip Rollano

Three Tales of Teen Pregnancy

By Jezaida Rivera

When we first became teenagers, my three best friends and I never believed that we would get pregnant in the near future. Even though there were a lot of young mothers in my neighborhood, we thought that it wouldn't happen to us because we were too smart.

But just for a good laugh we made bets on who would be the first to have a baby: Rayna, the tomboy, who beat up the boys who liked her; Gloria, the level-headed teacher's pet; Alexis, who loved kids so much she babysat for free; or me. They voted me to get pregnant first, because I was the most boy-crazy.

A few years have passed, and while I've been careful not to get pregnant, Rayna, Gloria, and Alexis all did. Here are their stories:

When Rayna was 15, she told me she was pregnant. I thought

it was a joke until I saw the tears in her eyes.

Rayna was dating Nate, an older guy with a bad-boy reputation. Before we knew it, Rayna lost her virginity to Nate. They had unprotected sex, even though Rayna knew she could get pregnant.

"I wasn't thinking about what would happen, only what was happening at the moment," she said. But after she found out she was pregnant, "reality kicked in," she said. "I thought 'What are we gonna do?'"

Rayna was scared to tell her mom. She thought her mom would be so upset and disappointed that she'd kick her out of the house. When she told Nate, he asked if he was the father, even though she had told him he was the only guy she'd ever had sex with. I guess that was his way of trying to get out of the situation.

After that, Nate didn't come see her or call her. When Rayna called his house, his mom said he wasn't home. When Rayna went to his hangouts, he wasn't there either. She felt used and alone.

Gloria didn't want a baby, but it was too late.

Rayna knew she wasn't ready for the responsibility of being a mother. If she wasn't responsible enough to protect herself, then she definitely couldn't handle being responsible for someone else's life. Rayna hunted Nate down to ask for money to get an abortion. She didn't want to tell her mom, who was against abortion. When she found him, he gave her $400 for the procedure, but he didn't offer to come with her.

I went with her to the clinic. I tried to tell her everything would be OK, but I knew she wished it was her boyfriend telling her that. She told me, "I was thinking to myself, 'Will I regret this?'" But she went through with it.

When I told Nate that Rayna had gotten the abortion, he decided to call her again. Eventually, Rayna got back with him even though he had ditched her when she needed him the most. When Rayna asked him why he avoided her when she was pregnant, he said he was scared.

Rayna said she took Nate back because he loved her. When I told her that I thought Nate was no good, she stopped talking to me for three months.

Later, when I asked her how she felt about having an abortion, she said it was the right choice. "I don't think I would be in college, be able to party, or be living with my mother if I'd had the baby," she said. Getting pregnant, Rayna said, "taught me a lesson."

I n the middle of high school, Gloria—the level-headed one in our group—started thinking about having a baby and moving out of her mom's house. She thought her mom was too strict. At 16, she decided to move in with her older boyfriend, who had his own apartment.

After a couple of months, his true colors came out. He expected her to clean, cook, and give him money for bills while she was working part-time and going to high school. Gloria realized that the relationship between them wouldn't work and returned to her mother. By then, however, she was 17 and pregnant. She didn't want a baby, but it was too late.

Her mother told her she would support her whether or not she had the baby. Gloria didn't believe in abortion, so, earlier this year, she gave birth to a girl. With her mother's help, Gloria finished high school and is looking into colleges. Although she says she wouldn't give up her baby for anything, she has some regrets.

"At first, I didn't want to have her," she said. "I can't imagine life without her, but I still wish I would've waited. I can't do things I used to do, like take a bubble bath or take a nap. I can't relax because I know that once I do, the baby is gonna start crying," she said. "People I called my friends don't come see me anymore 'cause [when I'm out] I'm always calling my house to see if the baby is OK. I think they see me now as an old person." She added, "I'm grateful my mother is helping me. I don't know what I'd do without her."

Rayna and Gloria both had rough times dealing with their pregnancies, but Alexis's story is the most dramatic.

Alexis fell in love with a boy named Stephon when she was 14 and he was 15. Alexis moved down South with her mom, and decided to have a long distance relationship with Stephon. A year later, Alexis moved back to New York to be with him.

When Alexis came back, she was devastated to discover that the guy she loved had been seeing someone else—and the other girl was pregnant. Stephon told Alexis that it was over; he didn't want to be with her because he was engaged and about to be a father. But Alexis wanted to be with Stephon so badly that she had sex with him. She got pregnant.

She had wanted to trap him; to have his baby so they'd always be connected. When Alexis told her father, he made her get an abortion. Stephon knew about it, but never came around. And soon, we heard that the other girl's baby wasn't even Stephon's.

At 17, Alexis got pregnant by Stephon again, still hoping to trap him. Her father decided that he couldn't make her get another abortion, so he helped her get an apartment. He asked Stephon to live with Alexis. He didn't want his daughter to walk around with a baby and no partner. Stephon agreed to move in with Alexis. What did he have to lose? He had been living with his mother and sharing a room with two sisters. Alexis's father was paying the rent, so Stephon would be living for free.

Alexis had wanted to trap him; to have his baby so they'd always be connected.

Alexis dropped out of school to spend all her time with Stephon. Stephon dropped out as well. (He was never really into school to begin with.) Neither of them was working.

As I mentioned, Alexis loved kids to the point that she baby-sat for free. But she told me that after being with her own baby for 24 hours a day, seven days a week, she lacked the patience that she once had. Alexis hadn't wanted to have any more kids after her first, but she got pregnant again. And again after that. She said she didn't want to take birth control pills every day. She didn't have information on other forms of birth control and Stephon didn't like to use condoms.

Stephon helped out with the first baby. But when the second baby came, he left all the parenting to Alexis. By the time the third baby was born, Stephon had checked out for good. He worked for about six months, but when he saw all his money going to diapers, formula, and bills, while his friends bought jewelry and new clothes, he quit. Alexis's father got tired of supporting Stephon and the babies so he sent Alexis back South to her mom.

When I asked her how it feels to have three babies at the age of 20, Alexis said, "It's hard. Sometimes I just wanna leave everything behind."

One time, said Alexis, "I left the girls [with my mother] for a couple of days to go party." She didn't tell her mother where she would be or how long she would be gone.

"When I went home, my clothes were in bags in front of the door," she said. "When I knocked on the door, my mom sent the girls out," Alexis said. "She was crying and told me we had to leave." Her mother kicked her out.

Now, Alexis lives in the projects down South and is receiving public assistance. Since the girls occupy most of her time, she never finished school. I asked her what she saw herself doing in five years. "I can't have any goals but to be a good mother," she said.

Obviously, my friends' lives have been shaped by their pregnancies. After going through an abortion, Rayna doesn't take the risk of pregnancy lightly. Sometimes she wonders what it would have been like if she had kept the baby and often feels guilty about her decision when she reads anti-abortion ads. Then there's Gloria, whose baby takes up much of her time, but she is still focused on her education due partially to her mother's support. Last is Alexis, who now has no education, no support, and three daughters.

My friends' choices have also shaped who I am today. I know that having a boyfriend doesn't necessarily mean having a baby. But at this point in my life, I avoid getting into a committed relationship because I'm afraid that what happened to my friends might happen to me.

If I got pregnant, I know that I would hate to make a choice between having a baby and an abortion. But faced with a decision like that, I think I would make the same choice Rayna did and have an abortion. Like Gloria's mom, I think that my mother would help me out if I got pregnant. But I wouldn't want to do that to my mother because my kids should be my responsibility, not hers. And as for how I relate to Alexis's situation, I just can't see having two or three kids.

To be honest, my mother has scared me into not wanting kids, telling me that having a baby now would ruin my life. I don't want to be responsible for someone else. I want to travel the world and that can't happen with a baby. But the biggest reason I don't want to have kids is because my mother told me that everything I put her through, my own children will put me through. And God knows, I've put my mother through a lot.

I want to be the kind of parent my mother was to me. Even though we never had much money and had our problems with each other, we never lacked love or friendship. If I have a baby, I want to be sure that both my partner and I are ready to be parents. I would like to provide a stable home. I don't want to be living from paycheck to paycheck. I want my child to have the best—financial security and a prepared, loving family.

Jezaida was 18 when she wrote this story.

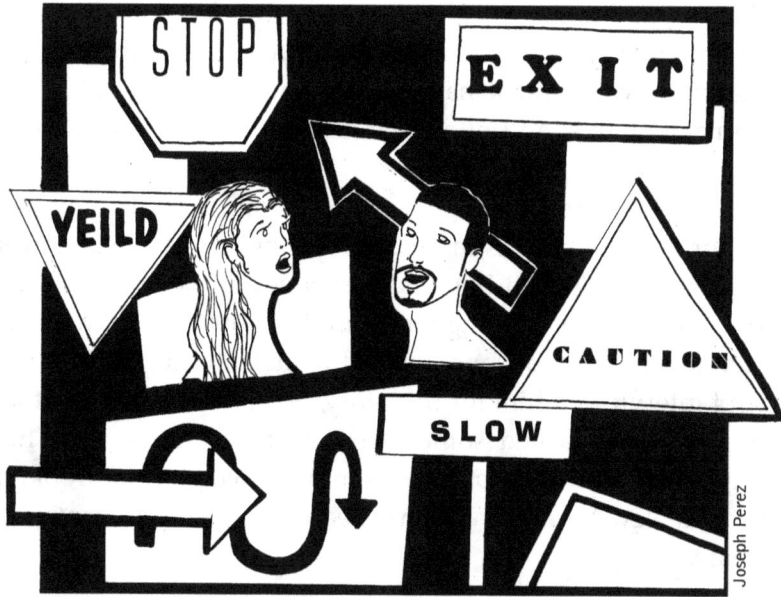

Joseph Perez

Getting Some (Answers)

By Lenny Jones

It's a Friday night, and you and your girlfriend or boyfriend have just come back from the movies. You have a romantic dinner at home (you just ordered Chinese), and you start critiquing the movie (especially the love scenes). Soon, you're kissing and touching.

One thing leads to another and soon you've got nothing on but your underwear. Of course you've always used protection before, but this time you realize that neither of you has a life preserver (a condom)! What should you do?

A. Stop.
B. Drive (or run) to the pharmacy.
C. Just say "Whatever" and get yours.
D. Create a homemade condom out of Saran Wrap.

Made you laugh with that last one, right? But, seriously, is there anything lying around the house that could substitute for a condom? I've found it hard to find answers to many sexual dilemmas like this, and often I've just been too embarrassed to ask for advice.

So I found a reliable source at The Door, a youth center in New York City, who was more than willing to answer my questions. His name is Rob Jiggetts. He's a sexual health counselor who will tell you everything you want to know. He really speaks our language (not that sophisticated medical terminology crap). When I interviewed him for this story, he made me feel comfortable, and even cracked some jokes. And he knows what he's talking about. Rob has a bachelor's in psychology from Brooklyn College in New York City and has been working at the center for six years.

Here are some of the questions that I asked, and his replies:

Q: What are some myths about sex you have heard from young people?

A: One myth is that a girl can't get pregnant if you're doing it standing up because the sperm can't move up the vagina. Not true. Those bad boys can swim very fast. Upside down, sideways—it doesn't matter. If you're not using any barrier or protection there, those boys will swim.

[I've also heard a myth about] douching afterwards, which means that a young woman will grab some water, vinegar, some Summer's Eve, and shoot it inside the vagina hoping to flush out the sperm. That's only going to piss those sperm off even more and they're going to swim up even faster. You're never going to catch them. As soon as they get away, those boys are gone.

(And actually, it's not good for girls to douche often. By shooting all those chemicals into the vagina, you're making yourself more susceptible to sexually transmitted infections.)

Q: One thing that I didn't know before coming to The Door is that you are supposed to press out all the air at the tip of the condom before you put it on so that the air bubble won't cause it to pop. Do you think a lot of people misuse condoms?

A: Yeah. A common mistake is to use oil-based lubricants like Vaseline or lotion. You shouldn't use those products on a condom. They will eat away at it, causing it to rip. Use water-based lubricants, like K-Y Jelly, instead.

Another problem is that people keep condoms in their wallets all the time. Wallets are tight and compact and will wear out the condom. Make sure that you don't overheat your condom. And don't put them in your back pocket. You're sitting, standing, sitting, standing, so you're like dry-roasting that poor condom.

If you have a condom dated 1987, you better throw that bad boy away.

And condoms have expiration dates. If you have a condom dated 1987, you better throw that bad boy away.

Q: Are condoms reusable, washable, or recyclable?

A: No. [Use a condom] once and once only. You weaken it by trying to wash it out.

Q: If a person doesn't have a condom at the time, can any household products (such as Saran Wrap, plastic bags, etc.) be used as a substitute?

A: Household goods in place of a condom? Na! Na! Don't try those things. Scratch that idea.

If you don't have a condom, I always suggest outercourse, which usually means mutual masturbation—touching each other, heavy petting, just as long as there's no exchange of body fluids. There are many ways to satisfy one's partner besides penetration, but you've got to use some creativity, some imagination, some fantasy. Penetration is not always the ultimate.

Q: If a guy is hittin' it through the back door (anal sex) without a condom, can she still get pregnant?

A: Pregnancy can still take place because the vagina and the anus are right next door, which means if the male ejaculates in the anus, you only need just a little drop to drip down and the vagina is right near by. Once those sperm get into the opening of the vagina, anywhere near the vicinity of the opening, they can swim up in there.

Q: Is it ever safe to go in without protection?

A: No.

Q: Can a girl get pregnant if she swallows sperm?

A: Na, 'cause we're talking about two different systems, digestive system verses your reproductive. But she can contract an STI if her partner is infected.

I just want to finish this off by giving a little tip for the guys and one for the girls.

Guys: Never let a girl talk you out of wearing a condom, even if she says she likes to feel the real thing. Is it really worth the risk of going blind, crazy, or even dying? Having a burning sensation every time you take a piss? (I didn't think so.)

Girls: The same for you. Don't let a guy get in you without a condom, no matter what he says. You have to be independent and carry your own!

Remember, don't get sexual health information from sources who are not reliable. Get information from people who know, from reliable Internet sites like plannedparenthood.org or sexetc. org, or drop in and talk to a counselor. And anything you're not sure about, don't be embarrassed to ask.

Lenny was 20 when he wrote this story.
He attended Parsons New School of Design.

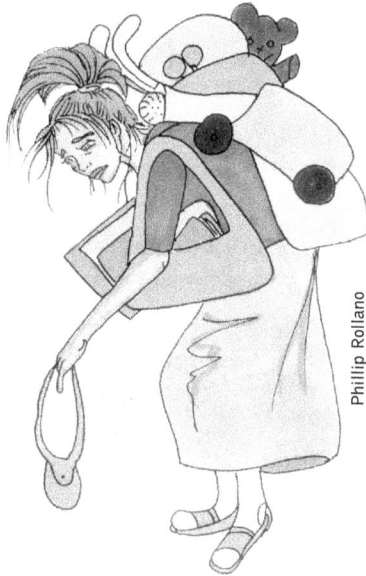

Phillip Rollano

Mom Wasn't Ready for Me

By Anonymous

My mom was only 16 when she had me, her first child. By the time she was 23, she had three little girls. I don't think she was ready for any of us. She needed more time to grow up and deal with her own problems. She didn't need the lives of three young girls adding to her own issues. But she went ahead and had us before she was ready. Now, partly because of all this, I'm in foster care.

My mom told me she had me so young because she wanted someone to love and to love her back. I understand the need to be loved, but if you want someone to love you, get a dog. Once you train that dog to love you, it knows nothing else. But a baby is not like that. A baby doesn't just give like that. A baby takes and takes and takes and takes. If you have a baby because you want to receive love, you're bound to be disappointed, and the baby will feel it.

I don't think my mom realized any of that. I don't think she realized how difficult it is to be a mom while you're still trying to grow up yourself. She hopped and skipped right over her childhood, and then she stumbled, and we, her kids, struggled with her.

By the time I was about 8, I already had too much responsibility. My mom supported our family financially, but she had me supporting us in other ways. It's like she was the working wife and I was the housewife.

If you want someone to love you, get a dog.

After school I would come home and do my homework, make sure my room was clean, and help my sister with her homework. Then, after the other kids were asleep, I was still up doing my chores. I'd clean the dishes, scrub the bathroom, and iron my baby sisters' school clothes. I would also get my grown mama's clothes ready for her to wear to work the next day.

Even the weekends weren't easy. On the weekends, I washed everyone's laundry. Now, I don't mind helping out around the house, but that was just too much. I feel like I missed my childhood trying to clean up after my family. But I didn't feel like I could say no, because if someone wasn't doing all the things I was doing at home, I might have gotten put into foster care much earlier than I did.

So now I have strong feelings about teen pregnancy. I think people should wait to grow up before they have babies. If you wait, you have more time to learn how to deal with stress without resorting to violence or neglect. You also have time to save money for a child, and get used to holding down a job. You'll be less likely to blame your children for opportunities you might miss out on. Having babies at a young age can make everyone in the family struggle more than they need to, especially the kids.

When I was picked to attend a conference on urban girls (which I thought should really be named "Ghetto Girls"), I looked forward to hearing the part about teen pregnancy. I thought that some of the speakers might be teen moms themselves, and some might have been the daughters of teen mothers, like me. I figured we'd all talk about teen pregnancy and how it had affected our lives.

But that wasn't what happened. Instead, everyone who went to the session on teen motherhood sat around listening to adults tell us about the teen moms they had interviewed. (Why couldn't those moms have just spoken for themselves?) But what surprised me the most was not that adults were doing all the talking, but that they spoke only about the teen moms, and not about the children of teen moms. Some of them talked about how it was nonsense that teen moms can't succeed in life. One spoke about a teen mom who, several years after having a child, was actually more successful in her career than her sister, who had not been a teen mom.

Of course teen moms can finish high school and work good jobs. My mom has a good job, and I'm proud of her for it. But what about the children? Will those kids get the love, care, and attention they need while their teen parents are busy trying to grow up and be successful? Right next door there was a talk on foster care, but not once during the teen parent session did I hear anyone talk about what can happen to the child of someone who isn't ready to be a parent.

It's like my mom was the working wife and I was the housewife.

There is a teen I once knew by the name of Shauna. She was someone who I felt was the perfect example of an unfit mother. Shauna had two jobs—a job which paid, and a job which didn't pay. Unfortunately, Shauna only took the job which paid seriously. Her other job, the job of being a mother, she gave only the slightest bit of time.

Shauna would wake up and get ready for the job that gave her the salary she wanted. Then she'd come home that evening to the job she didn't really care for, the job where she let herself be lazy—her job as a mother. If only she knew that her job at home was the most important job!

Shauna's precious little life at home, a 4-year-old boy named Leo, rarely got the attention and affection he needed, as Shauna was hardly ever home to give him motherly care. When she was home, she didn't want to be bothered with him. She was succeeding in the world, but she was neglecting her son. And what will happen to Leo as a result? Will he be able to grow up strong without the attention he needs?

The National Campaign to Prevent Teen Pregnancy says it will be a hard path for him. According to their 2004 study "Costs of Teen Childbearing," children of teen mothers tend to have more difficult lives than kids born to older parents. They are more likely to drop out of high school and earn less than the kids of older parents. They also suffer higher rates of abuse and neglect, and are more likely to go into foster care, like I did.

She had me before she was ready, and ended up giving me the same hard life she had.

But the problems don't end in childhood. The sons of teen mothers are about twice as likely to end up in prisons. Daughters of young teen moms are about a third more likely to become teen mothers themselves. (Which won't happen to me!)

So how could anyone, in good conscience, have a workshop on teen pregnancy and spend the whole time talking about how the teen mom can still finish school and succeed? When a child is born, I like to think that's one extra person who must be saved in this hard world. So thinking about the mother first is not something I tend to do. The first thing I think about is getting this child the love and care it needs. Why do so few other people think like this?

Too often, when we only worry about whether a young mother can still be successful in the world, we forget to ask if the mother can be successful at home. But we need to ask those kinds of tough questions when talking about teen pregnancy, questions like: Will the teen mother make sure that child is well protected? Is she financially able to raise a child? Has she had a chance to learn how to handle stress in healthy ways? Or will she abuse or neglect that child?

I know too many teen mothers who act the same way after they have a child as they did before they became parents. I've known some teen mothers who walk around in brand name clothes, while their children's clothes are raggedy and don't fit. It's clear to me they weren't ready to be moms—they still care for themselves way more than they care for their children.

My own mom truly loved me and wanted the best for me. She did not want me to grow up like she did. She wanted me to have things that she didn't have, and she wanted me to live a better life than she lived. But she wanted too much and too soon. She had me before she was ready, and ended up giving me the same hard life she had.

The author was 17 when she wrote this story.

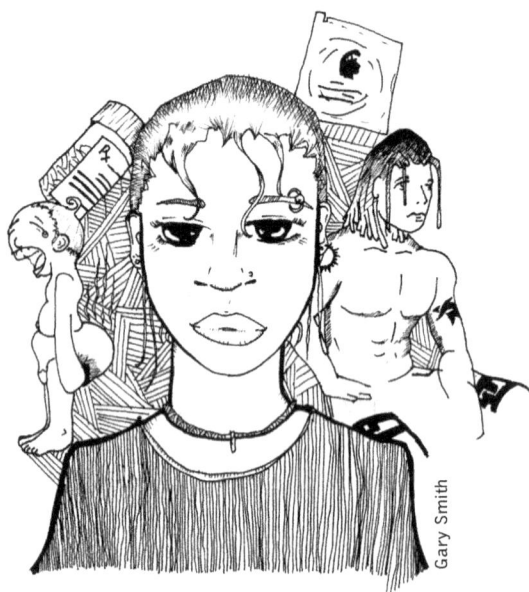

Gary Smith

The Morning After

By Anonymous

I'm a 20-year-old black female attending a university in the South. I first started having sex during my freshman year. I liked having casual sex, partly because I found on-campus relationships too complicated.

I recently met a guy named Dante. He had decent looks and a good sense of humor. He was in the Army, majoring in civil engineering at a historically black college nearby. He took pride in being a black man doing big things, and that was very sexy to me.

I'd been seeing Dante for a couple of weeks when I called him over to my apartment on a Friday night during booty-call hours—any time between midnight and dawn. I supplied the liquor and he hooked up the videos. I had a few drinks because I was feeling so antsy. I was soon buzzed.

We finished one movie and then started to watch a second.

It felt like we were waiting to devour each other. We never finished watching the second movie. I was prepared for the moment when we started to get into each other, and had the condoms by the bed.

Only, that night, Dante had a hard time keeping his erection. We tried putting on the condom, but he shrank again. That's when I made the decision that I later came to regret: I decided to start having intercourse without a condom. I figured we could put on the condom after he was able to stay erect.

Granted, this is very risky behavior because of the presence of pre-cum, which is semen that comes out of the penis before ejaculation. Pre-cum still contains sperm and can carry infections like HIV, syphilis, chlamydia, and gonorrhea.

That night I decided to take a chance because I was less concerned about pre-cum than about having no sex at all. Dante maintained his arousal and then entered me.

At this point, I thought about stopping and asking Dante to put on a condom, but I didn't. I was buzzed and I didn't want to break the rhythm we'd finally achieved. The night was finally taking off. I was caught up in the moment.

Sonya's eyes bugged out and her mouth fell open when I told her I let Dante hit it raw.

That is, until he let out an, "Oh damn!" We'd only been having sex for a few minutes. Dante pulled out and, with a look of mixed pleasure and fright, lay down beside me.

"I just came," he said, breathing heavily. I don't remember what he said after that because I was thinking, "I know you came quick. And possibly inside me." It seemed like he pulled out after he came, but I wasn't sure and I didn't want to ask. It felt like too hard of a question.

"Could I get pregnant from this?" I wondered.

"Are you on birth control?" he asked.

"No," I said.

There was silence. I was determined not to panic. I wanted to wait until I was a little more sober and could sort everything out. So I went to sleep and let him spend the night. With hugs and a kiss, we parted later that morning with an, "I'll be in touch." He sheepishly nodded and left. I knew I wasn't going to call him again.

I played the night's events back over in my mind. In my head were the excuses I'd heard from other girls who didn't think their risky behavior could get them pregnant: "It happened too quickly. He wasn't in long at all."

I remembered sitting through the health lectures at school and watching TV specials, thinking, "At this point, who doesn't know that unprotected sex can equal pregnancy or worse?" And here I was trying to convince myself that I couldn't be pregnant even though I'd just had unsafe sex!

I had homework to do, errands to run, and friends to catch up with, so I convinced myself not to worry. But I was two, maybe three weeks into my menstrual cycle, which is the time when women are most likely to get pregnant. Thoughts of my stupid actions and possible pregnancy seeped into my head while I was in my apartment, at the food court, in the library, and talking with friends.

I couldn't take a chance and wait to see if I was pregnant. I knew what I had to do. I would take the "morning after" pill— more appropriately the "up-to-three-days-after" pill.

One of my high school friends had a pregnancy scare a year ago and did a lot of research on emergency contraception, as it's called. She told me how it worked. I had 72 hours to take the pill—it's useless after that. The pill tricks your reproductive system into believing you're already pregnant. The body then builds a defense system to block a fertilized egg from setting in your uterus.

Even though I had a solution, I still wasn't clear about how to handle it. And I needed to calm myself down. So Saturday afternoon I talked to my friend Sonya. We'd talked about birth control before, so I thought she could soothe my anxieties by giving me informed advice and not judging me.

Still, Sonya's eyes bugged out and her mouth fell open when I told her I let Dante hit it raw. She told me that the possibility definitely existed that I could be pregnant; she said I should go to the school's clinic on Monday and ask for the morning after pill. But it was only Saturday and I worried about waiting two days. The more I tried to push negative thoughts out of my mind, the more they pushed back.

I'd assumed that if I had an unwanted pregnancy, I would have an abortion. I had no desire to be anyone's mother. Having a child would wreck my chances of achieving my goals. But now that the possibility seemed real, I worried I would consider abortion murder.

My worry was like a little snowball that grew bigger as it rolled down the hills of my mind. I regretted having unprotected sex with Dante and being at the mercy of the weekend. I spent the rest of the weekend doing homework, waiting. I just wanted to get to Monday, get my pill, and move on.

I swallowed the morning after pill and said, "Now do your thing."

At 8:30 Monday morning, I made an appointment over the phone with the student clinic to get the morning after pill. A million thoughts passed through my mind in the hour between the call and my appointment.

"Should I tell Dante what I'm doing?" I wondered. "And could I tell my mom?"

"No," I told myself. If I took the pill, I wouldn't get pregnant. I wouldn't tell Dante because we hadn't been a couple and didn't have a major emotional attachment. He hadn't even called to see if I was OK.

As for mom, I wanted her to think that I was safe. From this point on I knew I would be and didn't see any reason to upset her. It would be hard for me to forgive myself for disappointing her.

At the clinic, a nurse saw me first. While taking my blood pressure and body temperature, she asked me if the sex was consensual, if I'd failed to use a condom or if it had broken, and if I was on birth control. I said the sex was consensual. A few minutes later, Dr. M. entered.

Dr. M. asked me the same questions and recited information about the importance of consistently using condoms, the hazards of pre-cum, and the need to protect myself against sexually transmitted infections. Dr. M. said I should use birth control if I couldn't be counted on to use condoms regularly.

As she talked, Dr. M. bobbed her head back and forth with the authority of a judge with her gavel, saying, "If you keep this up, it's only a matter of time before you get pregnant."

I felt stupid having to listen to her speech. I hated feeling like I was a stereotype, one of too many black girls who can't remember to use condoms and end up pregnant.

Dr. M. gave me the first of the pills right there in her office with instructions to take the next one in 12 hours. I took the last pill at 9:30 that night in the library, well on my way into studying all night.

They were the smallest pills in the world, but they felt larger than the vitamin horse pills I take daily. I felt hopeful that the worst was over when I swallowed the pill and said, "Now do your thing."

Luckily, I didn't suffer any physical side effects from the pills. There could've been nausea, vomiting, vaginal spotting, and headaches.

My pregnancy problem was over, but I still had a lot of questions. Over the next few days, I tortured myself with conflicting thoughts about sex and relationships, and wondered if I'd ever be tempted to not use condoms again. I questioned if I should just have serious relationships and give up booty calls.

What hit me hardest about the experience was that I let my

desire for good sex get the better of me. Instead of putting off sex when things weren't working, I got caught up in the heat of the moment.

I realized that I still felt that sex is a beautiful thing; my desire is normal and won't shake. But I can control the situations in which I have sex so I don't do foolish things. I didn't want to slip up in my bedroom again. So I've resumed a healthy sex life. But I don't ever want a nightmare like the one I had over not using condoms.

Dante called me about a month after my pill drama. He talked to me like nothing had happened. I told him that I had to take emergency contraception. He sounded relieved that I wasn't pregnant. Then he admitted that he came inside me. Hearing him say that made me realize he didn't deserve me. I was right about my decision to take responsibility for myself.

My new partner is more considerate. We've had sex a couple times and he's as insistent about using condoms as I've become. Like me, he's scared of pregnancy and infections and wants to maintain his peace of mind. Looking back to that weekend with Dante, I was too antsy about having sex with him. Now I take time to enjoy the moment and remember to be safe.

The author was in college when she wrote this story.

What You Need to Know About Emergency Contraception

If a condom breaks or you have unprotected sex, it's still possible to protect yourself from getting pregnant by taking the "morning after pill," also known as emergency contraception (EC) or Plan B. Emergency contraceptives do not protect you from STIs (sexually transmitted infections).

You can use emergency contraception up to five days after having unprotected sex. However, it is most effective if taken within 72 hours (three days) after having unprotected sex. The sooner you take these pills, the more likely they'll prevent pregnancy. Emergency contraception pills work in a few ways. They can stop an egg and sperm from meeting, or stop the egg from attaching to the uterus so you can't get pregnant.

Short-term side effects may include nausea, fatigue, and breast tenderness. Your menstrual period may be temporarily irregular after taking EC.

Emergency contraception is safe, but it shouldn't be used in place of birth control because it's not healthy to take it often and it's not as effective as many other kinds of birth control. Even if you take it within three days, it prevents pregnancy only 75–89% of the time.

The cost of emergency contraception varies a great deal, depending on where you go and what services you need. Plan B may cost anywhere from $10 to $70. If you are under 17 and need a prescription, you will also have to pay for the visit to the clinic, which can cost $35-$250 depending on where you go.

If you're 17 or older, you can get EC at your local pharmacy or health clinic without a prescription. If you're under 17, you must first get a prescription for EC from a clinic or your doctor's office, or you can ask a friend or family member who is 17 or older to buy EC for you at a pharmacy.

To find a list of locations that provide emergency contraception, call: (1-888) NOT-2-LATE (1-888-668-2528), or visit

http://ECLocator.not-2-late.com

If you have other questions about pregnancy, or want to find a Planned Parenthood health center, go to www.plannedparenthood.org or call 1-800-230-PLAN.

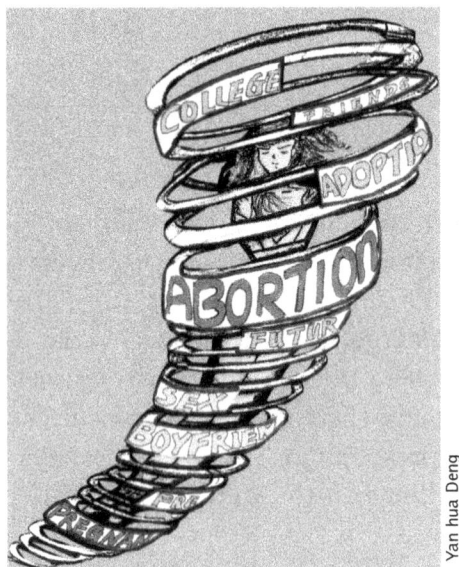

Yan hua Deng

The Right Choice for Me— for Now

By Anonymous

When I found out I was pregnant, I knew I was in for it. I knew it would be a hard thing to deal with and that I would never forget it. I was right. My mind keeps replaying that scary experience and my heart still aches when I think about it.

This is what happened. When I was 17 years old and two weeks away from being done with 10th grade, my old boyfriend called me. I say "old" and not "ex" because I always seemed to get back with him when he returned to the city during his vacations from college.

Our relationship began when I was in 9th grade and he was a senior. It started out slow. But, by the end of the school year, the relationship had become sexual. I didn't have a big problem with this. He was not my first; I'd had sex before. And I always wanted to see him.

When he called to say he was home from college, the topic of seeing each other came up. I said, "Sure. How 'bout this week?" I knew I had a half day coming up at school. When the day came, I had butterflies in my stomach. By the middle of the day, I was waiting outside my school. I pictured him picking me up in a little red sports car that was shiny and expensive. When he drove up, his car was little and it was red, but not new and not shiny. I joked with him about this. Then we were on our way to his house.

I knew that sex was on both of our minds but I didn't want to talk about it. I felt embarrassed after not seeing him for a while. In the car, we held hands and talked about school. When we got to his house, we just watched TV and laughed at dumb talk shows.

I had a few moments of panic, thinking about the possibility of being pregnant.

After an hour of flipping back and forth between shows, I felt a sexual urge that pushed me forward. I was a little scared but I definitely wanted to do this. We kissed a little and then we went to it. While it was happening, I was thinking two different things at once: "This feels right," and, "What the heck am I doing?" I thought it might not be a good thing for me because I hadn't seen him in a while. But I guess the "this feels right" took over because I didn't stop.

Afterwards, I felt fine. We hung around his house for a while and then he drove me back home. I wanted to see him again, but neither of us called the other. I'm not exactly sure why.

About two weeks later, I started to feel strange. My body was constantly aching and climbing stairs was harder than usual. I had a few moments of panic, thinking about the possibility of being pregnant. I didn't want that to be true, so I tried to block it out of my mind. But after I started getting sick every morning, my mom asked me if I thought I was pregnant. I said,

"Maybe." Then I said, "Yes."

My mom was very helpful about it. She didn't get mad at me. I was more upset than she was. I started to cry. I was so scared of what might happen. I didn't want to be pregnant.

We went to the doctor and I found out that I was seven weeks pregnant. The doctor asked me what I wanted to do. I told her I needed to think about it. I was shocked and overwhelmed.

I love children, but I knew that I wasn't ready to be a mother. I knew that my mother would help me as much as she could, but she has a job and would not be able to take care of a baby all day long. And I doubted that I would get support from the father. I didn't even tell him I was pregnant. I was scared that he would deny that he was the father and I didn't think I'd be able to deal with that.

I would also have to go to school in the last months of my pregnancy. My school is so small that everyone knows everybody else, and being the pregnant girl would mean I'd be teased and tortured. Besides, I had dreams of going to college. Having a baby would force me to rethink my future.

I love children, but I knew I wasn't ready to be a mother.

It was a short time before I told my doctor that I wanted to have an abortion. The thought of getting sick, of having a baby, of being pregnant at school made the choice clear. I was afraid, but I knew that it was best for me to have an abortion.

I talked about it with my best friends and they were mostly shocked at first, but then they wanted to talk about it and help me. Even after making the decision, I was still really crazed and nervous. My friends helped me calm down.

On the day of the abortion I woke up scared. At first, I didn't want to go, but my mom told me that I had made the right decision. At the hospital, my doctor calmed my nerves and told me what she was going to do. She gave me a lot of painkillers, but the procedure still hurt. I was mostly awake during it, though I don't remember thinking about anything.

Afterward, they put me in a wheelchair and took me into a room full of people who were recovering from different operations. When the nurse asked if I wanted anything, I said I wanted to go see my mom. I didn't want to stay in that room. It was too scary. There were too many other people around. I just wanted to see my mom and go home. When I finally did get home, I slept for a long time.

More than a year has passed since then. I still think about the abortion a lot. Sometimes I wish I'd had the baby.

I finally told my old boyfriend that he had gotten me pregnant. His reaction was just the opposite of what I thought. He said he would have helped me with the baby or at least would have liked to be with me when I had the abortion. I felt a little bad that I didn't tell him. But, at the time, I was really mad at him for doing this to me. I hadn't thought about his feelings that much.

I still think that it was best for me to finish school before having a baby even though I feel sad about the abortion. If I was out of high school, I think I would have had it. But school was much too important, plus I didn't want to sacrifice the freedom to hang out with my friends whenever I wanted.

Because of the pregnancy, I'm much more careful about sex and protection now. I started taking the pill even though I don't really want to have sex that much anymore. When I do want to, I will make sure I feel safe and happy with the person I'm with.

I want to have a baby when I meet the right man and it's the right time for me. But it's not that time yet.

The author was in high school when she wrote this story.

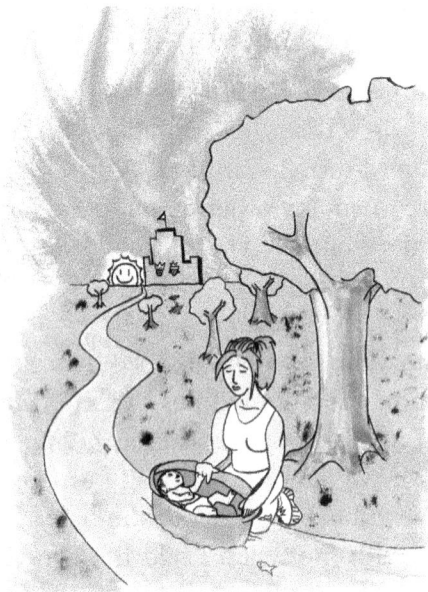

Andrew Rentoumes

A Family to Raise Her

By Jennifer Jeanne Olensky

It has been 11 years since I said goodbye to my daughter. As I sit here looking at her picture, I remember feeling as if all the glory of heaven was shining down into my heart and soul when she was born. This tiny miracle was the most beautiful child I had ever seen. Now, I think about how it all happened, and what led me to the choices I made.

Shortly after my 13th birthday, I went to live with my father. When I was very young, he had made me feel like "Daddy's little girl," showering me with love. But when I was 5, my parents separated, and my dad disappeared for three years. At the time, I believed his absence was my mother's doing, and hatred for her became embedded in my heart. I spent that time building my father up in my imagination. He was a king to me, he could do no wrong.

When I finally saw him again, my quest to live with him began. It led to bitter fighting between my mother and me, until the day she let go. When I arrived at Daddy's, I thought I had what I had wanted for so long.

I was wrong. My daddy loved me. He told me so every day. The only problem was his need for pills and heroin. Often we did not have food to eat. Eventually, he began beating me. He would punch me in the head and knock me to the ground. As I lay on the floor waiting for him to finish, he would kick me in the back of the head and legs. There were several times that I thought I would die. By the morning he never remembered.

I knew I had to leave, but I really had nowhere to go. My mother would hang up the phone upon hearing my voice, so I turned to my boyfriend, Alex. I was 14, he was 18. He snuck me into his house some nights. Not wanting to get him in trouble with his family, I would often sleep in his car.

Alex was all I had. He told me he loved me and I believed I loved him. For three months, I clung to him for my life. Then the police picked me up. After my first physical, I was sent to Rosalie Hall, a home for pregnant teens. That was the way I learned that I was pregnant.

When I told Alex, he said that if I didn't get an abortion, he was washing his hands of the whole situation. But I never even considered abortion. I wanted a family. At the time I had no one, and I guess I needed something to hold onto. When Alex told me he wanted nothing to do with a baby, I was upset, but also in denial. I didn't believe that he would be so cold. I thought eventually he'd come around—but he didn't.

The 30 other girls in Rosalie Hall, the aides who spent most of the time with us, the teachers, counselors, cleaning lady, and even the cook welcomed me. They tried to be like family, but they were not. I had lost everything. I felt alone and scared.

Alex still insisted he loved me, which gave me something to hold on to. He kept in touch until I was about three months pregnant. Then he told me he couldn't see me or call me anymore. He said it was only because he was pretending to see this other girl so that his family wouldn't find out I was pregnant with his baby. I was foolish enough to believe him.

For the next two months, I thought mainly about Alex. But after not hearing from him for all that time, I began thinking about my baby. The more I thought about it, the more I knew I needed to give my child a good life. The hardest part was realizing I could not. I was alone in the foster care system, but I wanted my child to have a loving, supportive environment with a mother and a father.

At five months, I decided to give my child up for adoption. I told my counselor, Stephanie. We spoke about it several times. I knew deep within that it was the right thing to do, but I decided not to tell anyone else. I knew the other girls would ridicule me, and the decision was hard enough already.

I knew I needed to give my child a good life. The hardest part was realizing I could not.

During the last few months of my pregnancy, Alex visited once and called twice. Each time he proclaimed his love for me. I believed all he said. I guess I needed to believe. Like with my father, in my eyes Alex could do no wrong. I spent every waking moment listening for the phone to ring, wishing he would call. Most nights I cried myself to sleep.

I felt alone and I knew, without a doubt, that my decision to give my child up for adoption was right. How could I allow a child to be subjected to the pit I had found myself in, abandoned by everyone I loved, and all those who claimed to love me?

When I was seven months pregnant I met Ann, a social worker with the adoption agency. She came to visit me several times. I told her I wanted my baby to have a good life. She did her best to assure me that everything would be fine.

Ann presented me with files of different families. Eventually, I chose a couple who had been together several years. She was a college professor, he a lawyer. From their file, I felt confident that they had a strong sense of family, with a marriage built on mutual love and respect. I knew they were the ones.

On September 28, my labor started. On September 29, I arrived at the hospital at 9:30 p.m. I was alone, scared, and in a world of pain. Looking back with the faith I have now, I believe God was with me, not only in those final hours of my pregnancy, but every step of the way. I cannot understand where all my strength and energy came from if not from God.

On September 30, at 1:46 a.m., I looked into my daughter's eyes, and love, joy, and happiness overwhelmed me. In the midst of all life's tragedies my heart was singing. For the first time in my life, I felt true love. Over the next two days, I spent every possible moment with her. I never wanted to forget. I never wanted that feeling to fade.

The adoption agency was supposed to pick her up on the third day. I was not ready to let go. I asked for three more days. Ann, the adoption social worker, was reluctant at first, but gave in.

The evening before I was released from the hospital, Alex came to see us. I had called to inform him of her birth. I suppose he wanted to satisfy his curiosity. He held her and fed her. When he said goodbye, he left in tears, never voicing his feelings. It was devastating. Part of me wanted him to say, "OK, we are going to keep her!" But I knew it would not happen.

For the next few days after I left the hospital, I was living close by so I walked over about four times a day to see my baby. She was extremely quiet. I never heard her cry. She would let out a small noise, then put her fingers in her mouth. She fussed a little when hungry, but as soon as she heard my voice, she became quiet and alert.

It had only been a few days and I felt so connected. "How can I do this?" I thought. I asked Stephanie, my counselor, what would happen if I changed my mind.

"Foster care," was her response. "You did not apply for mother-child placement. There are waiting lists."

I thought about it and knew it would be wrong. She deserved an immediate welcome into a warm, loving environment, not the uncertainty I would face. Besides, I wanted her to have a permanent, stable home, and that was something I knew at the time I couldn't provide.

The morning Ann came to get her, I had time for one feeding. As I held her, I spoke to her, studied, rocked, and hugged her. After some time I settled her into the bassinet and rubbed her back as she fell asleep. Kissing her head, I said goodbye. It was so hard to leave. I began to feel numb, just going through the motions, trying to stay strong.

As the adoption papers were explained to me, I sobbed, unable to stop.

Then we went to Stephanie's office with Ann and Sister Diane, who was supposed to witness and notarize the signing of the adoption papers. As the adoption papers were explained to me, I sobbed, unable to stop. Sister Diane said, "That's it! I will not notarize these papers. You are keeping your baby." Then, Ann put the pen in my hand. That shocked me, and suddenly I stopped crying and signed the papers. I quietly walked back to my room and stared at the wall.

I don't remember much of what happened over the next several days. As I slowly resurfaced, I thought about the couple, my daughter's parents. Instead of thinking about my loss, I was able to imagine their joy as they set their eyes upon their child. I shared in their happiness and trusted that they would take this truly amazing gift and nurture her, love her.

Like I said, all of this happened 11 years ago. I have some pictures, and a five-page letter her parents sent me. My daughter's parents wrote that I was their angel sent from heaven. They said I was a special person with the capacity to love in a special way. I also sent a letter to them and one for our daughter when she is older. I know I will see her one day, and hope to develop a relationship then.

I did what was right and do not regret it. In giving her up, I gave two loving people the family they longed for, my daughter a chance to thrive, and myself the opportunity to grow and become the person I am now. I think of her on a regular basis. She is a part of me. Although I cannot see her, the love for her in my heart continues to grow.

Jennifer wrote this story in a parents
workshop at **Represent** *magazine.*

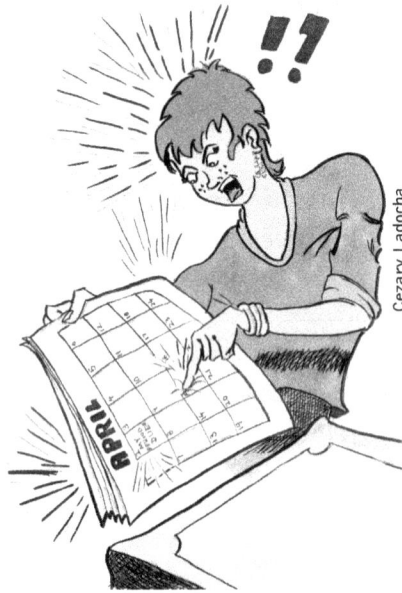

Cezary Ladocha

Stressed About Sex

By G. Santos

One evening in April, my close friend Samantha sent me an instant message.

"I need to talk to you," she wrote.

"What's up?" I typed back.

Samantha said that she'd had sex with her boyfriend. He'd used a condom and withdrew before he came. Afterward, Samantha was scared that she might be pregnant, even though she'd had safer sex.

She told some of her friends what had happened, and one of them told her she could be pregnant. She was nervous and needed to talk to someone else. So she instant messaged me. Thanks to the brochures I read on birth control, I knew that if used correctly, condoms had a high success rate.

"If you have sex with a condom and it doesn't break, then

you're fine," I wrote her. She was reassured, but not for long. Samantha called me the following morning.

"Hello?" I answered in a drowsy state.

"I'm still worried that I might be pregnant," she said.

I thought Samantha was being unnecessarily anxious about the situation. I told her to ignore her friend's comment. I kept on repeating, "You used the condom and it didn't break." The chances of her being pregnant were quite small.

A lot of girls aren't ready for how they'll feel after having sex. Even those who use protection still experience anxiety just over the act of having sex. I have other friends who've had similar stressful experiences. My friend Janice always used protection when she had sex with her long-time boyfriend, but even a condom wasn't enough to keep her from worrying.

I wanted to take back those stupid few seconds of pleasure, because it wasn't worth my present anguish.

"I always think that even 0.00001% of sperm can get into me and get me pregnant," she once told me. "It's really scary when the stress about getting your period mounts up."

She and her boyfriend dealt with that stress by deciding to focus more on alternatives to sexual intercourse, like just spending time with each other or foreplay. Foreplay can involve hugging, kissing, touching, and rubbing, among other things.

I sympathized with Samantha and Janice because I'd had a pregnancy scare. But unlike them, I was scared because I hadn't used a condom during sex.

I was messing around with my boyfriend. Things got hot, and he entered me. But then he quickly withdrew without ejaculating, since neither of us had a condom. I thought I was pretty safe, even though girls can get pregnant from pre-cum, a fluid that guys emit before ejaculation that can carry small amounts of sperm.

The possible consequences of my actions didn't hit me until weeks later, when I was late for my period. My cycle is usually irregular, but I couldn't help worrying that I might be pregnant. Days went by slower than usual because I was constantly aware that my period was late. My imagination ran ahead. I started to think about how my boyfriend and I were too young to be parents, and imagined my father disowning me if I told him I was pregnant.

After a week and a half of waiting, I was in the pharmacy. I hadn't meant to, but I walked through the birth control section and wondered if I should buy a pregnancy test. I confided in my older cousin, who has two kids, and she listened to me patiently. She told me to wait a few more days to see if my period came before taking any action.

If Samantha was constantly worrying every time she had sex, then I thought she shouldn't be having sex.

But after almost two weeks, I didn't know what to do. One night, I broke down and cried. I wanted to take back those stupid few seconds of pleasure, because it wasn't worth my present anguish. Finally, more than two weeks after it was due, my period came. I was so relieved.

After that incident, I promised myself to never let a guy enter me unless he was wearing a condom. I didn't want to succumb to a moment of weakness again, where I'd forget about using a condom because I was so overwhelmed by my physical desire.

Samantha sounded like she had far less to worry about than I had. I believed she was so anxious partly because she wasn't emotionally ready to have sex. The same thing had happened before. The first time she had sex, she and her boyfriend used a condom but she was still nervous. She became so worried about being pregnant that she told her mother. Surprisingly, her mother comforted her and told her to wait and see. Her period soon came.

If Samantha was constantly worrying every time she had sex, then I thought she shouldn't be having sex. I told her during our phone conversation that I didn't think it was worth worrying for days on end over a few moments of pleasure. Samantha agreed with me that sex wasn't worth the constant anxiety. She said she discussed the issue with her boyfriend, and he said he wouldn't mind taking a break from sex. So they decided to do the abstinence thing for now.

It's often said that people should be "ready" before they have sex. I've learned that being ready means accepting that sex can be stressful, whether it's safer or unsafe. Still, there are ways to ease anxiety about sex. It's important to get information about safer sex from trustworthy sources like Planned Parenthood. Another good source for information is a health teacher or social worker/guidance counselor in your school. They can also refer you to different clinics and health services available to youth.

Once you feel more informed, it's easier to enjoy it when you're using condoms or other contraceptives. And if you feel that you're not ready, that's perfectly fine too. By practicing abstinence, you're at 0% risk of getting a sexually transmitted infection or getting pregnant. No matter what your decision is, it's important to be aware of the realities of having sex.

The author wrote this story when she was 17.
She graduated high school and went on to college.

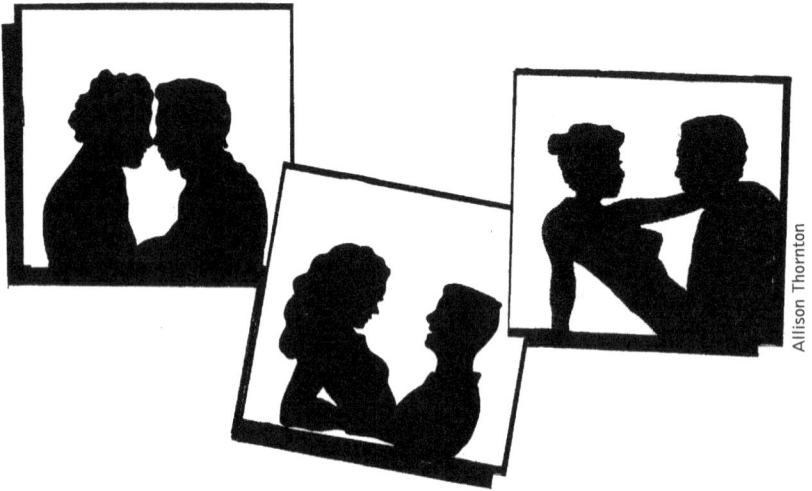

Allison Thornton

There's More to Sex Than Sex

By Anonymous

Humping, fingering, jerking off, rubbing, petting, licking, sucking, stroking, first base, second base, third base, foreplay, kissing, hugging, necking, making out....Call it what you want, there is a whole other world outside of sexual intercourse.

"People do a lot of crazy stuff before they do it," said David, 17.

But why not do the crazy stuff *instead* of doing "it"? Especially if you don't have a condom, you're afraid of pregnancy, AIDS, or nasty things like genital warts—or if you're just not ready. People often overlook things like kissing, hugging, even holding hands.

"Anything can be erotic and enormously satisfying," said Andy Humm of the Hetrick-Martin Institute. "Sex is more than intercourse. It's more than doing the deed: The thing is in, the thing is out." Humm recommends that teens use their imaginations. There are many ways of expressing yourself sexually other than intercourse.

"Humping" is about the closest you can get without putting yourself or your partner at significant risk of catching a sexually transmitted infection (STI) or getting pregnant. That's when two people rub their pelvic areas together, simulating intercourse, but the penis does not penetrate the vagina. It can be done with or without your clothes on (although without clothes you have to be careful no semen or vaginal fluids are exchanged). People also use their hands to stroke, finger, and "jerk" each other. This is also known as mutual masturbation.

There are still some small risks that come with these alternatives. Even without having intercourse you or your partner can contract chlamydia, herpes, or pubic lice (crabs), for example, just through genital contact. What about HIV, the virus which causes AIDS? "Theoretically, if you rub too hard, there is a risk," said Teri Lewis, director of the AIDS and Adolescents Network of New York, "but people always have these 'What ifs?'" Any cuts, open sores or conditions such as poison ivy might pose a small risk if you choose to engage in mutual masturbation because they are potential passageways for infection.

'People do a lot of crazy stuff before they do it.'

There have been studies claiming that about 25% of all teenagers have engaged in anal sex, often to avoid pregnancy or preserve their virginity. But anal sex is not a safe alternative since there is a higher risk of catching HIV even with a condom. During anal sex, there is a greater chance that the condom will break and that tissue will tear even if you don't see any blood.

The risks of STIs and unwanted pregnancy can be avoided if you choose an alternative to intercourse. Michael has done some "other stuff" because he did not have a condom, but he adds: "If we had a condom, we would have done it."

If you're not ready for intercourse, but you think that you might be ready for some of the alternatives, there are some other things you should think about as well. "You have to ask yourself, 'Can I handle this?'" says Lewis. "'Do I trust this person? Can I speak to this person?'"

Some people can't trust themselves; once they get started, they can't stop themselves after a certain point. For some people, only intercourse counts as real sex. Still others aren't ready for what experts call "outercourse" either, or don't want to engage in any type of sexual activity until they are married. "There's no rush," said Ana, 17.

> **There are many ways of expressing yourself sexually other than intercourse.**

You have to decide for yourself what you think is right for you. Whether you choose to have intercourse, outercourse, or to remain abstinent, the most important thing is to talk about the decision with your partner.

There might be a point where you would like to stop. Say you don't want to do anything beyond French kissing, for example. According to Lewis, the two of you have to work that out together—ahead of time: "You have to decide that 'We won't get further.'"

But, what if your partner disagrees with you? "Ask yourself the hard question, 'Is this the relationship that I want?'" Lewis cautions. "If you can't reach compromises about this, then you probably can't reach others."

The author wrote this story when she was in high school. She went on to receive a BA in Art History and work in marketing.

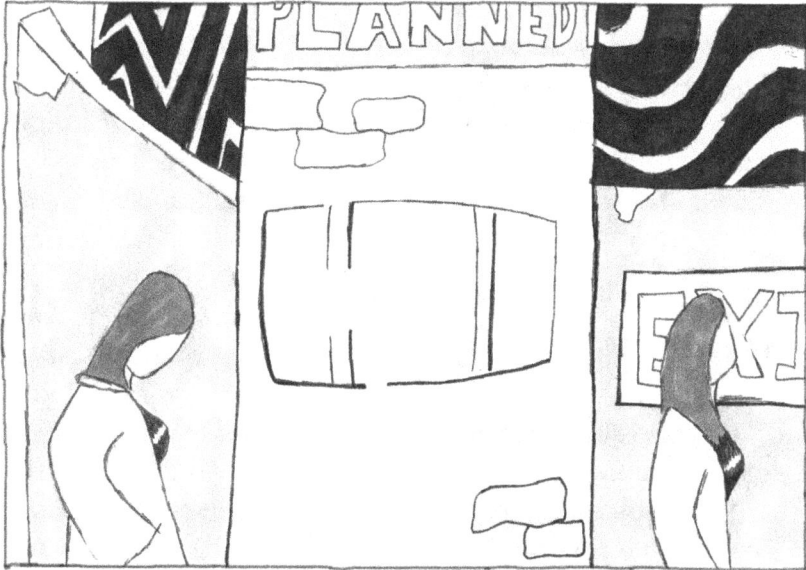

Steven Mattor

A Difficult Decision

By Anonymous

During my time in foster care, I have lived in several homes with teen parents. The most memorable teen mom was only 16 when she had her first child, and was getting ready to turn 18 when she had her second. The only people she could depend on were her social workers, and sometimes not even them. She had no family and the fathers of her children did very little to help her. She was very much alone, struggling to raise her kids.

I swore that I was going to be nothing like her. I was going to finish school and get a job before even considering having a child. That was when I was 14. I had never been in a relationship with a guy, so I figured that getting pregnant at an early age would not happen to me.

Shortly after my 14th birthday, I began going out with a boy for the first time. He was friends with some of my friends, and was older—17. We had an off-and-on relationship that didn't involve sex, at least not for a couple of years. Most people assume that being in a relationship as long as ours without sex would take a huge toll on the guy, so I kind of thought that if I didn't eventually give him some, he'd leave me. Soon after I turned 16, we said that we loved each other for the first time and decided to start a sexual relationship.

I thought that if I didn't eventually give him some, he'd leave me.

At first I didn't think that having sex was going to change our relationship, but after a while it did. I think because I lost my virginity to him, it brought us closer together, even though sex isn't all that it's cracked up to be. See, I let TV and movies influence my thoughts about sex. They make it seem like it's this wonderful thing, and that it's all glamorous. Sure, it's OK, but it's also very weird. It feels funny, the positions are funny and it even smells funny. I don't understand why people exaggerate about it so much.

Anyway, my boyfriend and I didn't really talk about it, but we ended up using condoms for birth control. Even though I had never taken any sex education classes at that point, we just had the common sense to know that protection was the best thing for both of us. So every time we'd have sex, we used a condom. Except for that one time.

Summer started. Things were going well between my boyfriend and me. Then, as the summer continued, I began to notice some changes in my body. I thought it was because of stress, but decided to go to the doctor anyway. That's how I found out that I was three weeks pregnant. I didn't expect to hear that—my period was only a day late, so when the doctor told me the news, I started laughing. I thought she was joking. She gave me this look and said, "Seriously, you're pregnant." I still didn't believe it, not until she gave me some information about abortion and adoption. She told me to read it and come back in two weeks with a decision. I had to decide whether to keep the baby, have an abortion, or have the baby and give it up for adoption. This would become the hardest two weeks of my life.

When I told my boyfriend I was pregnant, he was more shocked than I was. He asked me what I wanted to do, and for some strange reason I said I wanted to get an abortion, even though I wasn't really sure. It just seemed like the logical thing to say. My boyfriend didn't have any objections. He said I should think of my future, which was true, since most likely I would be the one raising the child.

Then, the next weekend I was watching TV when I turned to a show called *Eclipse of Reason*. It showed actual footage of a woman getting an abortion, and interviews of two women who said they were hurt mentally and physically from having abortions. By the end of the half-hour, my stomach was turning and I was in tears. The program led me to believe that if I went through with an abortion, I was a bad person. So my mind was set: I wasn't going to get an abortion. I felt as if I had made a big decision, but reality would soon wake me up.

When the doctor told me the news, I started laughing. I thought she was joking.

I was looking through a bunch of papers that I got from the Internet and from my doctor about abortion. The factual information I read there was surprising, and very different from the TV show, which I now think was created not to give an accurate account of abortion, but only to persuade women not to have them. The information from my doctor and the Internet reported that the mental and physical complications from abortion are extremely rare.

Then I began thinking of the teen moms I knew, and especially those whose kids later ended up in foster homes without them. I realized that *Eclipse of Reason* showed women getting abortions, but it didn't show young women struggling to raise kids alone, with no money, no support, and no job.

I began to think about all the things I wanted to do with my life that would be hard to do if I had a baby. I wouldn't be able to go to college full-time. If I found time to get a job, I wouldn't get to keep the money for myself. I would have to buy baby clothes, milk, and diapers, and pay for a babysitter just to leave the house.

And having a kid at my age would not just be unfair to me, it would be unfair to the child, who would grow up without stability. He or she would be subjected to an unprepared mother and an environment where nothing is certain. The child would have to deal with the stress of having her mother struggle and do her damnedest just to keep a roof over our heads and food in our stomachs. I suspected I would make a good mother someday, when I had a steady job and a roof over my head. I also knew that now wasn't that day.

But I still didn't want an abortion. The thought of it was scary, and I wondered if it was wrong. So I thought briefly about adoption, but didn't like the idea of carrying something for nine months and becoming bonded to it as it gets big, and then having to give it away. So instead of deciding what to do, I didn't decide. I went past my two-week deadline to go to the doctor and to let them know what I wanted to do. Finally, I realized time was running out.

The day I decided to call Planned Parenthood for an abortion was the longest day of my life. I tried calling from the time I woke up until about 1 p.m., when I finally got through. I told them that I wanted to make an appointment. The woman on the other end asked for what, and for some reason the word "abortion" could not come out of my mouth. When I finally said it, she gave me a date to come in: the next day. I was hoping to have a couple of days to collect myself before I had the operation.

The next morning my foster mother and boyfriend went with me to the doctor. When I got there, I saw many women of all different ages, all waiting to have an abortion. One girl I met was 14 and was also having her first abortion. Another woman was 30 and already had two kids and had had two abortions before. We passed the time talking and watching TV.

When I finally made it into the operating room, I lay on the table. After that, all I remember is praying to God, asking Him to let me make it through OK. About 20 minutes later I woke up and started crying. Then I went home. All day, as I dealt with the aftermath of the abortion—mostly bleeding and cramps—I thought about my decision. I pictured myself with and without a baby. I thought about whether I was going to hell or not because of the abortion.

To this day, almost a year later, I still think about what my life would have been like with a baby. For one, I probably would be raising it alone, because my boyfriend and I broke up, though we're still great friends. For another, I probably wouldn't be going away to college this fall. And though sometimes I still have mixed feelings about abortion, for the most part I'm glad I made the decision to have one.

I think it's irresponsible to just say that abortion is bad without also showing how hard it is to raise a child before you're ready.

Not too long ago I was looking through the TV guide and saw that show *Eclipse of Reason* coming on again. I thought about the message that show was trying to get across—that abortion was evil and that it would scar a woman for life if she had one. I think it's irresponsible to just say that abortion is bad without also showing how hard it is to raise a child before you're ready.

Yes, it's a bad idea to become pregnant when you aren't ready to be. And people should do everything they can to prevent unwanted pregnancies. But I think abortion only becomes bad when women see it as something as simple as brushing their teeth in the morning. If they say, "Oh well, I'm pregnant again, so I'll just get an abortion," they're using it as a form of birth control, and I think that's wrong. But once a woman is pregnant, she is the one who should decide what to do, because she is the one who will live with her decision. And believe me, making that decision is hard enough without people telling you what to do.

Not too long after I had the abortion, people found out. They made sure they expressed their opinions. Quite a few were angry with me. They had the "How could you do that?" attitude. A few others had the "You made the right decision, but…" attitude, and still others congratulated me and said they were surprised at how someone my age could make such a big decision. I do feel like I made a big decision. In some ways, it was one of the most difficult decisions I've ever made.

The author was 17 when she wrote this story.
She later attended college.

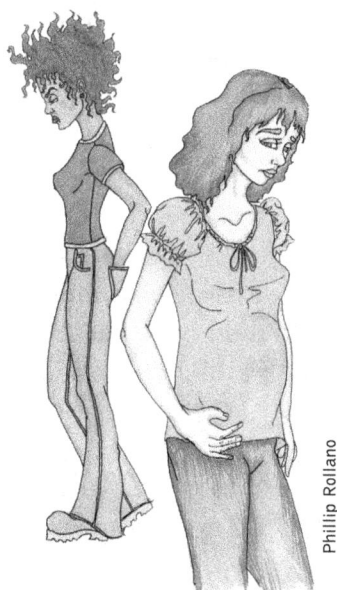

Phillip Rollano

Keeping My Baby

By Anonymous

When I first meet Tee-Tee, I had already heard rumors that she was nosy. I lived in a group home, which is a kind of dormitory for foster kids like me, and Tee-Tee was a new staff member there. She had a reputation for telling other residents your business, so at first I was not nice to her. I would roll my eyes at her for no reason, and I wouldn't talk to her.

But after a while I started to think she was nice and sweet. During school vacations, Tee-Tee would take us to the movies, or drive us to Blockbuster to rent DVDs. I started to think, "Why do I always listen to what other people say? Why don't I give Tee-Tee a chance?"

As time went by, I became close to Tee-Tee. She was always there when I needed someone to talk to about my problems, or issues with my mother. Tee-Tee felt close to me, too. She even told me that she wouldn't leave her job until I finished high school. She wanted to look out for me and that made me feel special.

I may not have listened to anyone else, but I always listened to Tee-Tee. I knew that anything she told me was for my own good. There was only one thing I didn't listen to her about.

Tee-Tee always talked about how important it is to have safer sex. She said that it's easy to become pregnant or get an STD (sexually transmitted disease). She always said that she does not believe that girls should have babies, because they are only babies themselves. She said that having a baby puts your whole life on hold. It makes it harder to finish high school and reach your dreams.

Tee-Tee knew that I was having sex, so she set up a doctor's appointment for me to get birth control pills. I took the pill for one day, then I threw them all away. A resident at my group home gave me at least 20 condoms, but I did not use any of them, either. Even my boyfriend wanted to use condoms, but I didn't want to.

You're probably wondering why I did that. I think my mind was playing tricks on me. I would never have said that I wanted a baby, but I think a secret part of me thought that if I had a baby I would have something to love, and later it would return that love to me.

At the time, I was feeling very lonely. My mother was not talking to me, and my boyfriend was thinking of leaving the area for college. I did not feel like I was being loved by anyone that much. I just wanted love so badly. A part of me thought that if I had a baby, I would have the kind of love I wanted. I did not really sit down and think about the whole thing carefully.

Then the drama happened. My period was a week late. Suddenly, it scared me to think that I might really be pregnant. All the time I'd secretly wished for a baby, I wasn't thinking about the reality of it.

When I told Tee-Tee that I needed a doctor's check-up, she

immediately suspected something. She asked, "Are you pregnant?"

I said, "No."

Then she asked, "When was your last period?"

I told her I needed to go to my room to check my calendar, even though I knew very well that I was late. When I came back, I decided to tell her the truth. If I was pregnant, I needed prenatal care so that the baby could come out healthy.

I told Tee-Tee my period was late and she asked me if I'd had sex without condoms. At first I didn't answer her. I felt ashamed. Tee-Tee said, "Tell me the truth, did you?" I shook my head no. She started talking about why it is so important to

A part of me thought that if I had a baby, I would have the kind of love I wanted.

use condoms—a conversation we'd had many times before. Now I felt bad that I hadn't taken her advice. I knew how much Tee-Tee loved and cared for me. I knew that she wanted the best for me. I felt so upset thinking that I might be pregnant.

Eventually, I went to the doctor to take a test, but they told me that I would have to wait a few days for the results. I had been worrying for days, and I had to know now, so I bought a pregnancy test.

As soon as I got to the house, I took off my coat and went straight into the bathroom with the pregnancy test. After I took it, all the other girls huddled in the bathroom waiting to see what the result was going to be. There were two pink lines. That meant that I was pregnant. I was shocked. All of a sudden I started to scream.

Tee-Tee was on duty, but was about to leave. When I went to her, I had this funny look on my face, and she asked what was wrong. I said, "I took the test. Do you want to see it?" I felt sick as I said it. When Tee-Tee saw the two pink lines, her face fell. As she went to her car and drove off, I started crying. I had let her down. I was so upset about what Tee-Tee thought, I was not noticing my own feelings.

About two days later, it hit me. I was pregnant. I was really pregnant. I realized that if I had a child, my life would never be the same. I was thinking: "How am I going to raise a child in the foster care system? Will I be a good mother? Or will I be like my mother?" My mother used to always put me down and call me all kinds of names. I did not want to be that kind of mother.

I knew I wasn't ready to be a mom yet. After all, I was only 16 years old. I want to hang out with my friends, go to parties, and graduate from high school on time. With a child it would be much harder for me to do anything.

I knew I didn't have to be a mother at all. I could get an abortion or give the child up for adoption. But I thought that would haunt me for a long time, and I felt like I'd had enough hurt in my life. I think every time I would see a little baby I would cry, or wonder what my baby looked like. It would just be too much to live with. So, after thinking real hard, I made up my mind to keep the baby.

When I made this decision, Tee-Tee started acting distant and saying things that upset me, like how she didn't understand why babies have babies. When I told her that I would be able to know the sex of the baby by the end of June, she got mad and said, "That is not cool." Her whole attitude made me upset, because we had been close.

And it wasn't just Tee-Tee. Everyone I knew seemed upset. I let down my mother, my boyfriend's mother, and some of my close friends. Everyone I knew thought that this would never happen to me. They expected more of me. I had wanted to get pregnant so I could feel loved, but I felt more alone than ever.

After a while, I started having weird dreams about being a bad mother. In the dreams, I would see myself abusing my child. I also had dreams that I had a miscarriage, and that I gave birth to a retarded child. I started to get frightened. I needed someone to talk to, so I went to Tee-Tee, even though things were weird between us.

When I started telling Tee-Tee how scared I was, she explained why she'd been acting strange. She told me that she loved me and she really wanted to see me go on to college. It hurt her to know that, at 16, I would have to stop focusing on myself and my education and focus on a child instead. She had tears in her eyes as she explained these things to me. Seeing how much she cared for me, I started crying too.

After that, I told Tee-Tee that even though I had decided to have a baby, I was still having mixed feelings. I could no longer concentrate in school—in class, all I could think about was, "How am I going to take care of a baby?" Tee-Tee said that even though she was not happy about the whole baby thing, she would support me no matter what I did.

I hope I'll be a good mother, but at 16 it's hard to predict what you're going to be like for the next 18 years.

Talking to Tee-Tee made me realize that she gives me the kind of love I need—the love of a mother for a child. I know that a baby can't give me that. As a mother it will be my job to attend to the baby's needs, not the other way around. I understand that the child will come first now.

Soon, I will be moving to a maternity shelter, which I am not at all pleased about. It means I will have to leave the group home that I've been in since I was 13 years old. I'll be leaving everything I know—my neighborhood, my friends, and staff like Tee-Tee. Nothing in my life will be the same.

I know my relationship with my boyfriend will change, too. We will not be able to go out and do things together like we used to. Instead, if we want to go anywhere we will have to pay for a babysitter. And most of our attention will not be on each other, but on the baby. This might put a lot of stress on our relationship.

I still don't know if I'm doing the right thing, but I'm keeping the baby because I think it would hurt too much to give it up.

The Morning After

I hope I'll be a good mother, but at 16 it's hard to predict what you're going to be like for the next 18 years. I do know one thing for sure: If I could turn back time I never would have gotten pregnant. I would have taken the birth control pills and used the condoms.

The author was in high school when she wrote this story.

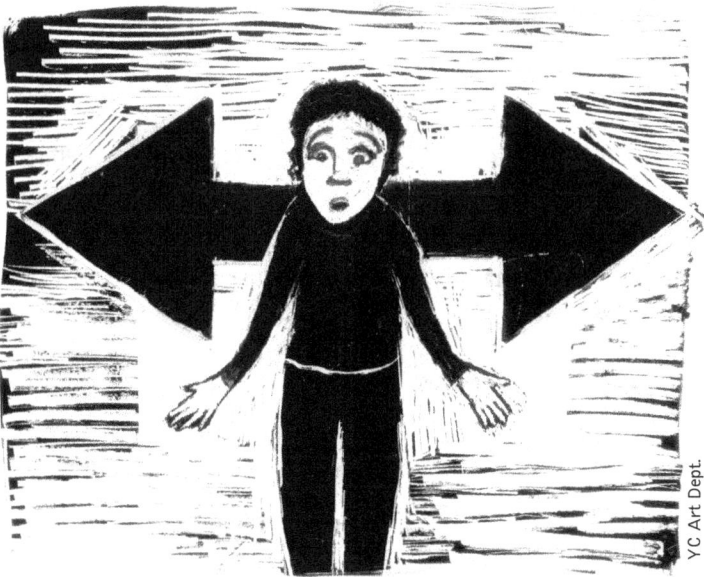

YC Art Dept.

A Choice I Couldn't Make

By DeAnna Lyles

"Are you hungry? Do you want a plate?" my boyfriend's mother asked one summer day.

"Nah ma, don't give her a plate. She's going to go home and make a pizza and then order Chinese food," my boyfriend interrupted. It was true. I had been hungry all the time lately and had gotten into the habit of eating four meals per day. My boyfriend's mom looked at me suspiciously.

"Are you pregnant?" she asked.

"Wow," I said as I laughed nervously, shocked by her question and unable to say anything else.

She shook her head. "I hope y'all use condoms," she said as she walked out of the room. As she turned the corner, my boyfriend hit me on the arm.

"Why would you laugh? Now you're going to have this lady

thinking you pregnant!" he yelled. "Well, are you?"

"I don't think so. I should be getting my period in a few days," I said.

But the suspicion grew. It went from my boyfriend's house to the very household where I lay my head. There is a belief in my family that dreaming about fish—any type of fish in any way—means that someone in the family is pregnant. That week, my mother dreamt about all types of fish swimming around in the big blue ocean. She asked all our female family members if they were pregnant—they all said no—and I was the only person left to ask.

It was an early Saturday morning and the sun was shining its brightest, blinding me even through my covers. All of a sudden, I heard my door being opened so forcefully it slammed against the wall with a big bang. I felt the covers being snatched from

I never thought that I would end up pregnant at 14 years old.

my body and straight ahead stood my moms, the fairest and scariest of them all to me. I barely had a chance to open my eyes before she started pointing her finger at me.

"Wake up!" my mother yelled. "I got a bone to pick with you."

I stumbled from my bed to the bathroom like a drunken monkey, but before I could relieve my bladder, my mom threw a small box at me. I was shocked by what I saw laying on the floor next to my foot; a pregnancy test. When I looked back up at my mom, she stood with her hands on her hips, tapping her foot, a devilish look in her eyes.

She said I had to take the test now, whether I wanted to or not. She made me keep the door open because she thought I might put water in the cup instead of my urine to mess up the test results. I didn't think I was pregnant, but everyone else's suspicions had me spooked. While I sat there and waited for the results to come back, I was scared. I prayed that it would be negative. My mother was the first to read the pregnancy test. When she announced it was positive—I was really, truly pregnant—I felt numb.

After that, she made me take three more tests. She just couldn't believe it kept coming back positive. Well, I couldn't believe it either. Each time another test came back positive, my eyes got wider and wider and my heart felt like it was coming to a stop. I never thought that I would end up pregnant at 14 years old. I wasn't sure if I should be upset or happy. I was just really confused.

My mother was upset, but not like I expected her to be. "Tell me what happened. It's OK. I'm not mad at you, I just need you to talk to me and explain."

"I don't know" I replied, as the tears came pouring down my face.

"How long have you been sexually active?" she asked, her face as serious as it had ever been. Her eyes were fixed on me.

"Since around my birthday. That's about four or five months now," I said, still crying my eyes out.

She took a deep breath and continued questioning me.

"Have you been using protection? I mean like every time?"

"Yes, Ma. We used condoms every time. That I promise you."

"Then how is it that you ended up pregnant?" she asked, starting to get angry.

"I don't know, Ma. We used condoms every time! It may have popped and neither one of us knew. I don't know." I wanted to walk away from her and the whole situation, but knowing that I couldn't, I just continued to cry. She said she understood that I was young and that mistakes do happen. But now, she said, I had to decide what I wanted to do: keep the baby or get an abortion. She said I had two weeks to tell my boyfriend and make my mind up.

A couple of days later I went over to my boyfriend's house to deliver the news. As I approached him, he could tell something wasn't right.

"What's wrong with you?" he asked with a deep voice.

"Umm, I think I'm pregnant," I told him. His mouth dropped like a dog in a cartoon. His entire mood and body language changed. He started pacing back and forth, scratching his head, and talking to himself.

"What do you mean you *think* you're pregnant? Either you are or you're not," he said furiously.

"I'm pregnant, OK? I took four pregnancy tests the other day with my moms. I'm letting you know so we can decide something before it's too late," I said.

"So, what the hell you telling me for? That's not my baby," he said as he walked out of the room, slamming the door.

As his words really started to sink in, I became hysterical. I didn't understand why he would say that. We'd been together for almost nine long months, and I loved him with everything I had inside. My eyes filled with tears, and my heart rate increased, making me feel like I just ran from my worst nightmare. When he re-entered the bedroom, about 45 minutes later, he realized the condition I was in and apologized. He held my hand and looked me in the eyes.

"Yo, to be honest with you, I'm not ready for a baby," he said. "We only 14 and still got our entire lives ahead of us. My moms still does for me, and with a baby around she won't do as much for me anymore." He told me that it was truly best if I did get an abortion for both our benefits, but said the decision was up to me.

I still couldn't get my feelings straight. For the next four or five days I struggled with the decision. I wanted to keep the baby because it was a living, growing human being inside of me. I felt the baby expected me to nurture it and bring it into this big world. At the same time, I was still a baby myself. With no independence, money, or work experience, I had no real way of supporting a child. I knew my moms would help me out, but it would have seemed like her child and not mine, since I wasn't capable of handling motherhood on my own.

I still had dreams and goals; I wanted to graduate high school, go to college for forensic science, and find a job and a place of my own. I doubted I could accomplish those things with a baby. If I had a child, there would be an endless amount of things that should have been, could have been, but probably would never happen. Still, I couldn't stand the idea of an abortion. Weighing my choices while time ticked by was driving me insane. As the end of my mom's two-week deadline neared, I was still unsure.

"So you know tomorrow is the deadline, right? Have you made a decision yet?" my mom asked nonchalantly like it was your average decision.

"No, I haven't," I replied back with attitude.

"What the hell are you waiting for?"

"I don't know. It's a hard decision for me. I want to keep the baby because it's mine. But then I'm not sure because I want to graduate high school, and then probably go off to college. I just don't know what to do."

"Well, it doesn't matter. I made the decision for you," she said. "You're getting an abortion."

I was immediately upset. I replied, "So what was the purpose of giving me time to think about it, if you was still going to decide for me?"

I felt the baby expected me to nurture it and bring it into this big world. At the same time, I was still a baby myself.

"I can't let you wait until you're five months along or further, so I made the decision for you and the decision is final. No more debates." She acted like it didn't have anything to do with how I felt. She already had my appointment set up and everything, I just had to show up. When my mother told me this, I felt like throwing up. I was upset at how easily she made a decision that would have such a huge effect on me. But, at the same time, I was a little bit grateful because if I had to decide on my own, I didn't think I'd ever make up my mind.

The Morning After

After that, everything seemed to happen really fast. I was scared. I had never even been to a gynecologist, so just the thought of the procedure had me terrified. Both my mom and dad came with me to the clinic. I was happy that they supported me, but upset that my boyfriend wasn't there, too. I really needed him to comfort me, but he told me that he just didn't want to go.

The clinic looked like any other. It had a very small waiting room, and a long hallway with plenty of doors. I waited a long time just to be escorted to another waiting room with other females changing into their gowns. All of us were getting abortions. After talking to the other girls there, I realized I was the youngest one. Everyone else was between 18 and 22 years old. They all had their boyfriends with them, and here I was with my mommy and daddy. I felt ashamed. I was still practically a baby.

After another half hour of waiting, my name was called, and I was escorted to the operation room. There was a bed with stirrups that I was supposed to put my legs through as I laid on my back. They hooked me up to a machine that would put me to sleep. The last thing I remember was the doctor telling me to count backwards from 100. I only got to 75 and I was out cold. When I woke up, I was still heavily drugged. I felt like I had to pee really badly, but I really didn't. I was bleeding, as if I was having a heavy menstrual cycle.

It was summer time, so I spent the next week cooped up in the house, in pain. It wasn't so much physical pain, but internal, emotional pain. I was angry and depressed because I knew I killed something that had been in the process of growing into something precious and worth loving. It took a long time for the emotional pain to subside but I eventually felt better. Re-entering normal life after being cooped up in the house for so long felt weird, but refreshing. It was good to get back to the basics of my life.

The whole experience changed my relationship with my boyfriend, with myself, and with others to come. I realized that, although neither my boyfriend nor I was responsible enough for a baby, I showed more maturity than he did. I was ready to deal with the situation and continue on with life as best as I could. But my boyfriend did what most males do in such situations: He ran. He thought he was grown enough to have sex with me, but he wasn't grown enough to accept that I was pregnant and he was the father. Soon after the abortion, we realized that our relationship wasn't going anywhere and we broke up.

Even though my life didn't have a dramatic outward change, I changed completely as a person. I decided to focus on myself more because I realized that I had been so wrapped up in my boyfriend's life that had I forgotten who I was. I had to sit back and really get to know myself again. And after the abortion, I didn't want to have sex because

Even though I was highly against abortion, I still got one.

I feared the same thing would happen again. It took me almost a year before I became sexually active again, and he's the only guy I have been with since.

Even though I was highly against abortion, I still got one. I'll never say that I agreed with my mom's decision 100%; I didn't. I wanted to make the decision on my own. However, I thank my mother for helping me through the ordeal. She made me look at my future, and realize that a baby would hold me back.

I'm still uncomfortable with abortion and consider it generally bad. But, in my situation, it was the best choice out of the bad options I had. I was so young, and there was just more in store for me than to have a baby. If I'm meant to have kids, I will one day. But hopefully I will have accomplished most of the things I set out to do first.

DeAnna was 18 when she wrote this story.

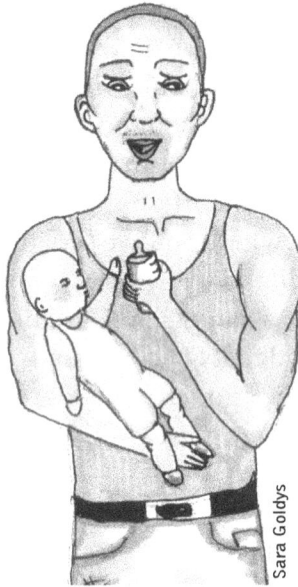

Sara Goldys

Why I Always Use a Condom

By Anonymous

It was raining outside and our plans were squashed. My girl-friend Kimberly and I had nothing to do. "Let's watch some TV," she said to me, but I had other plans. Little did I know they would lead to my biggest mistake.

We were alone in her house on that fall day five years ago. Her parents were at work. Sex wasn't anything new to us—we'd been steady lovers for almost a year. My plan was working to perfection when Kimberly stopped me.

"Do you have a condom?"

I told her I didn't.

"I don't want to have sex if you're not protected. You never know what could happen."

I told her not to worry, that it was no big deal if we didn't use a condom this one time. So we had sex. It was fun and made us both feel great. But the pleasure we had that one afternoon couldn't compare with the pain that followed in the months to come.

Kimberly didn't get her period. After a visit to the doctor, she found out she was pregnant. She went crazy. She was crying, almost shaking. She talked about running away from home. When I told her that was a stupid idea, she began to scream that she was going to tell her mother.

I pleaded with Kimberly not to do that. We were only 14 and just starting high school. I didn't think telling our parents would help—it would only get us in more trouble and they would probably make us break up. Kimberly agreed not to tell as long as I made the arrangements and paid for the abortion.

I told her not to worry, that it was no big deal if we didn't use a condom this one time.

It took two months to get the money together. Those two months were the worst of our lives. Kimberly was suffering emotionally and physically. She was depressed, vomiting, and had a headache every day. She had sudden mood swings and was growing quite distant. I was missing a lot of school and doing everything and anything to make money—odd jobs, gambling, robbing, stealing, lots of things I'm not proud of.

January came and, with it, the abortion date. When I woke up that morning I was nervous and jittery. I just wanted the ordeal to end. We planned to meet at 1 p.m. at the doctor's office. At 2:30 I was still waiting. At 3 p.m. I finally called her house.

"Meet me down the block from my house," she said. Now I knew there was trouble. I got there in about a half-hour and asked her where she had been. "I felt sick," she said. I offered to get her an appointment the following day, but she screamed "No!" She told me she woke up scared, couldn't take it any longer, and told her mother everything.

Her mother blamed me for what happened. "It's all his fault," she said. As horrible as it sounded when Kimberly told me this, her mother was right. It was my fault.

Kimberly's mother prohibited her from having the abortion. I was off the hook—I didn't have to pay for it. All I had to do, Kimberly said, was stay away and pretend I never knew her. If I didn't, her mother threatened to tell my parents about the situation. I had no choice but to follow the rules.

As the weeks went by, I was dying to know how Kimberly was doing. Even though we weren't talking, I still loved her. I began to spy on her. I'd wait for her across the street from her house. I'd hide in the bushes or sit in a parked car. Sometimes I'd follow her and I began to notice that she was getting bigger. She was going to have a baby—my baby! I had to talk with her. When I saw her go out to the store one day, I stopped her.

> *I began to notice that she was getting bigger. She was going to have a baby—my baby!*

"How are you?"

"Fine."

"Listen—you're having my baby. I think I should be a part of everything going on now."

"No, my mother and I agree you shouldn't be around. I don't want you around and I hate you!"

I could tell she wasn't really turning on me, just following her mother's orders. I was shocked and hurt, but there was nothing I could do.

"Goodbye!"

In the months that followed I lost all contact with her. It was May and school was nearly over. I should have been happy, but on the day vacation began I found out from a friend that Kimberly had gone into labor. I raced to the hospital.

"It's a boy!" I screamed in the hallway outside her room. I wanted to see my child, but her mother wouldn't allow me in. How could she do that? How could the hospital allow it? I argued, but it was no use.

I went to see Kimberly the night she got home from the hospital. Except for the hair and eyes, the baby looked exactly like me. I felt the joy of birth. Shortly afterwards her mother made me leave. On the way down to the bus I was jumped by three guys—friends of Kim's mom—who told me to leave Kimberly alone. "Never come here again or we'll kill you!"

I finally told my father everything and, even though he was upset and disappointed, he agreed to help me. After weeks of negotiations, Kimberly's mother agreed to visitation rights. Twice a month.

It was obvious whenever I visited that her mother was still angry. Two months after the baby was born they moved to Florida. They were gone for a month before I even found out.

I never stop thinking about what happened. And although I'll never give up responsibility for my son or be ashamed of him, I will always know that a mistake caused all this. We should have used a condom that day. Not only to protect ourselves, but to protect everyone around us who was affected by our behavior. My girlfriend became a mother at 14 and had to leave school. Her life was ruined and mine was changed forever. Had we been responsible that fall day five years ago, things might have worked out better.

In the last three years I've probably spent ten days with my son. I bounce him on my lap and play airplane with him, but he doesn't remember me and he doesn't call me Dad. Will he ever acknowledge me when I'm older? Will he ever understand?

The author was in high school when he wrote this story.

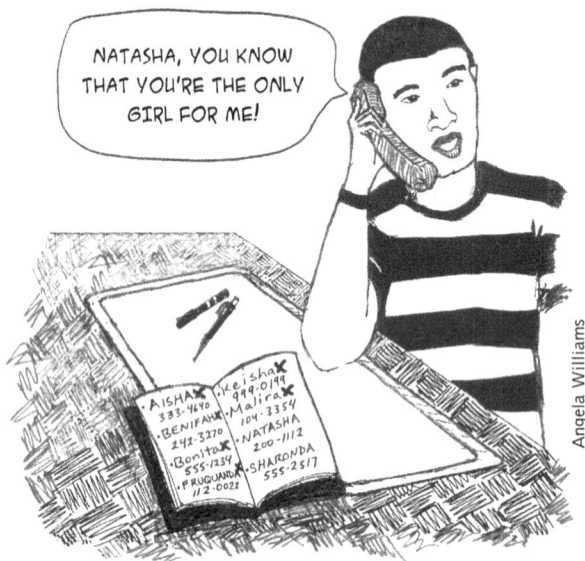

Angela Williams

If You Believe These Lines, Check the Price of Pampers

By Frank Jones

You're about to have sex and your boyfriend or girlfriend says, "I don't have protection but we've known each other since we were 3, so you know you ain't gonna catch nothing from me."

You try to avoid it by saying, "On TV they said the best sex is with a condom." Your boyfriend or girlfriend answers back: "You watch too much TV. If the TV said jump off the roof are you going to listen?"

Well, what can you say if you're in this position?

Dr. Mark Wade, medical director of the Cumberland Family Health Center in Brooklyn, New York and Segrid J. Renne, a health educator at Metropolitan Hospital, offer some suggestions on what to say when you hear some common "lines."

"I wanna get the real feeling out of it. I don't want no rubber."

Dr. Wade advises you say this to your partner: "Having sex with me is the real thing. If we're doing this right I'll make you forget about the condom."

Renne added, "If he really cared about his girlfriend he would consider her health and her future if an unwanted pregnancy occurs."

"If you make me use a condom, I'll leave you."

"Bye," Dr. Wade suggested, "No condom, no coochie."

Renne commented, "If he entertains thoughts that he will leave her then he really doesn't love her. All he cares about is the sexual act. Furthermore, he's not taking any precautions to protect himself against STIs."

"Yo baby, I love you and the whole nine, but I can't put it on because it don't fit."

"One size fits all. It could fit over your head," said Dr. Wade.

"Try filling it with water and see how it expands," suggested Renne.

"God made man and woman, not man and condom."

"God made man with the ability to think and to be responsible for his thoughts, words, and deeds, which includes protecting other people and himself from sexually transmitted infections. The condom is a contribution to the preservation of man's well-being," said Renne.

"You can't get pregnant. It's your first time and a virgin can't get pregnant."

"Of teenage girls who decide to have sex without the use of a condom about half of them get pregnant within the first three months. About one fourth get pregnant the first time," Dr. Wade responded.

"If a guy ejaculates and is not using a condom or any other form of contraception, the possibilities of the girl getting pregnant are high [whether or not it is your first time]," answered Renne.

"You can't get pregnant if we have sex standing up."

"Do you think the sperm is going to spill out? Do you think the sperm knows the difference if you are lying down or standing up?" asked Renne. "You can most definitely get pregnant if no contraception is used."

Dr. Wade replied, "It's not whether you're standing up, sitting down or laying down—it's whether you're inside or out."

"Don't worry, you can't get AIDS from a virgin."

"You can get AIDS from anyone who's infected," said Dr. Wade. "[Besides], you never know whether that person is a virgin or not."

"You can't get AIDS from me. Don't I look clean and healthy?"

"You can't see the AIDS germ. No matter how clean you look, or how you smell, AIDS is on the inside not the outside," Dr. Wade said.

"You may be a carrier and don't even know it," answered Renne.

"If you really loved me you'd have sex with me."

A good response, according to Dr. Wade, is: "If you really loved me, a statement like that wouldn't come up to pressure me. If you really loved me you'd make sure that you're protected and I'm protected."

The point is, there's a way to respond to every argument. If you can't think of one on the spot, quit while you're ahead; just say no. You don't have to have sex. It's better to wait until you're both mature and responsible enough to take the steps to prevent unwanted pregnancy and STIs.

Frank was 15 when he wrote this story.
He later became a karate instructor.

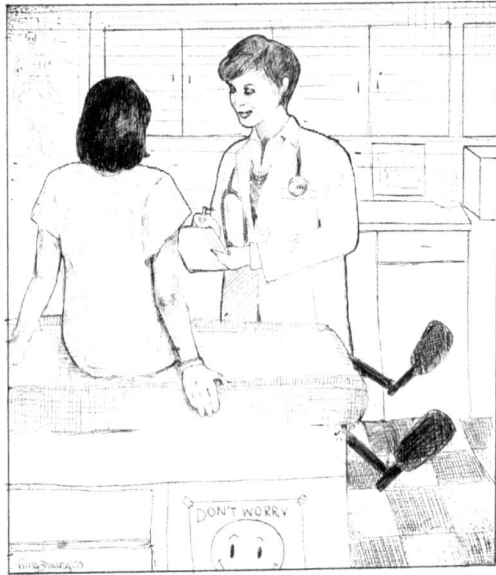

Qing Zhuang

Back in the Stirrups—Again

By Madeleine Gordillo

The birth control pill is an extremely effective way to prevent pregnancy—if it's taken every single day. But a lot of girls are afraid to get a prescription for the pill because of one big, scary roadblock: the visit to the gynecologist. To help relieve some of the anxiety, I'll explain the exam step by step. (It's still not the most pleasant thing in the world, but it's good to know what you're getting into, right?)

Your visit to the gynecologist begins like any doctor's appointment—you fill out forms about your medical history and your reasons for being there. There are many clinics where you can get exams for free, but you may be required to show identification.

At the clinic, you may be asked for blood or urine samples to test for pregnancy and infection. At some clinics, you speak to a counselor before getting examined by a doctor or nurse practitioner. The counselor, or sometimes the practitioner, reads your form and may ask for more information. (For example, if there is diabetes in your family, she'll ask which family member has it.) She will also ask why you are there and if you have any questions. If you came for something specific, like birth control, or to find out if you have a sexually transmitted infection, you should tell her that.

After the counseling session, you go into an exam room, where you are asked to take off your clothes and change into a paper robe. The exam table has metal hoops, called stirrups, attached to the bottom corners.

The examination begins with a breast exam. The doctor will open your robe and tell you to place both hands behind your head. Using the flat side of her three middle fingers, she'll feel for any abnormal lumps in your breasts and armpits. The doctor should also teach you how to examine your own breasts so you can do it between doctors' visits.

Many people fear it will be painful, but if you relax and don't tense up, all you should feel is a slight pressure.

Next comes the pelvic exam. This is when the practitioner asks you to lay down and put your heels in the stirrups. They keep your legs spread apart enough so that the doctor will be able to examine you properly.

The doctor will check the outer surface of your vagina to make sure everything looks healthy. Then she inserts the speculum, an instrument used to hold the walls of the vagina open so the doctor can see inside. The doctor will gently insert the speculum into your vagina. Once it's in place, she will open the mouth of the speculum. Many people fear that this will be painful, but if you relax and don't tense up, all you should feel is slight pressure.

The doctor will check the walls of your vagina and the opening of your cervix for any abnormalities (redness, inflammation, cysts, unusual discharge) that could be signs of infection or disease. If you have any questions about your reproductive organs or about what the doctor is doing, you should feel free to ask them during the exam.

Next, the doctor will insert a long Q-tip into your vagina to get some cell samples. (You might feel some "poking" at this point.) This is called the Pap smear, or Pap test, and it is done to test for warning signs of cancer. If you are sexually active, she will take another sample to test you for gonorrhea and chlamydia. This lasts about a minute. Then the doctor closes the speculum and eases it out.

Next, she changes her gloves and spreads lubricant on one or two of her fingers and puts them inside your vagina to feel your cervix and internal organs. You will feel a little pressure at this point. With her other hand, the doctor will press down on your lower abdomen to feel your uterus and ovaries. She does this to feel for any abnormal swelling, tenderness, or lumps.

The doctor will probably spend a few minutes discussing your exam with you when she's done. You will be told if anything abnormal was found during the exam, such as inflammation of the vagina, any unusual lumps, or discharge. The doctor might prescribe something for you or tell you that you need additional tests. Don't expect the results of your Pap smear and STI culture right away. That usually takes a few days. If anything irregular shows up in those test results, she'll contact you. If you don't hear from her, and you weren't told to call for the results, then everything's fine.

To stay healthy, doctors recommend that everyone have a physical exam every year.

Madeleine was 17 when she wrote this story.
She went on to college at Syracuse University,
where she received a BA in International Relations.

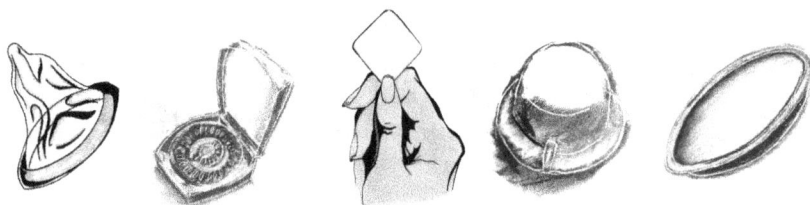

All About Birth Control, Right Here

By Rasheeda Raji and Kymberly Sheckleford

You must have heard it time and time again, but we're going to let you know one more time: abstinence, not having sex, is the only 100% sure method of avoiding pregnancy and sexually transmitted infections (STIs), including HIV, the virus that causes AIDS. But if you do decide to have sex, protect yourself and your body by knowing how to get and use condoms.

On the next few pages, we've provided information on both the male and female condom, which are the only two contraceptives that can prevent STIs. We've also explained how the pill and other female birth control methods work. By using condoms and birth control together, you reduce two risks at once: the chance that you'll get an STI and the chance you'll have an unwanted pregnancy.

Because you are putting your body on the line for someone else, consider talking to your partner about birth control and condoms before you start messing around. Get familiar with one another's sexual history. Share your feelings and concerns about sexual activity. You want to make sure that you are making a decision that you won't regret later.

If you become sexually active, you're exposing yourself to a whole new range of possible medical conditions. It's more important than ever to maintain your health. If you're a woman, get regular gynecological (GYN) examinations and STI tests. If you're a man, get tested regularly for STIs.

How to Use a Male Condom
(as demonstrated on a banana)

1. Use a new condom every time you have sex—before the penis gets anywhere near any body opening.

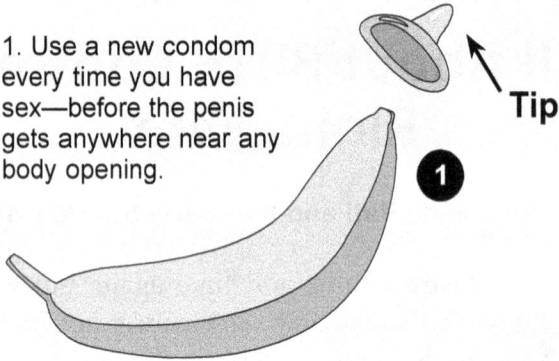

Tip

1

2. Make sure the rolled-up ring is on the outside. Handling the condom gently, pinch the tip so no air is trapped inside, and allow room for semen if you come.

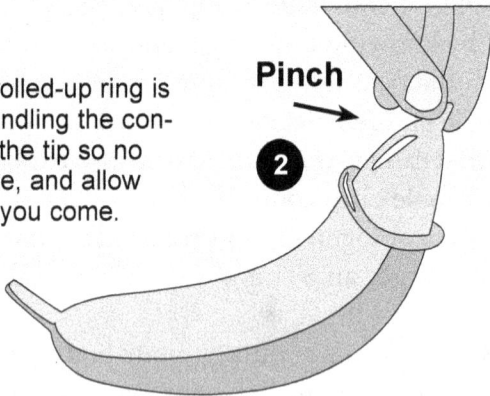

Pinch

2

Women can get pregnant from pre-ejaculate fluid (pre-cum), and both men and women can get STDs from skin-to-skin contact. Check the condom's expiration date and open the package carefully, since teeth or fingernails can tear the latex. Put the condom on as soon as the penis gets hard. If the penis is uncircumsized, pull back foreskin.

3. Hold the tip while you unroll the condom all the way to the base of the penis.

If it doesn't unroll, it's on backwards. Throw the condom away and start over with a new one.

Make sure that it fits and isn't loose. Experiment with different brands to get the right size.

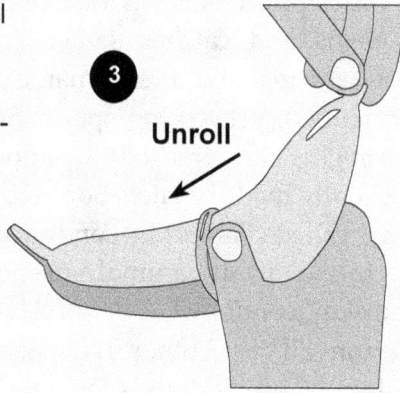

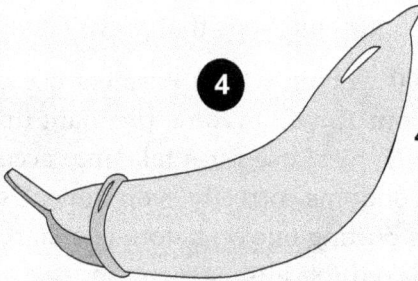

3

Unroll

4

4. You're ready.

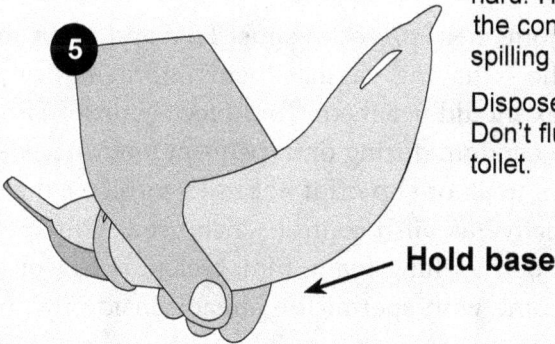

5. After sex: Pull out slowly while you're still hard. Hold the base of the condom to avoid spilling semen.

Dispose of it properly. Don't flush it down the toilet.

5

Hold base

THE CONDOM

Description: A cover that fits over the penis and catches semen (cum) before, during, and after a man ejaculates (cums), preventing sperm from entering his partner's body. Condoms are usually made of latex. Some condoms, called "lambskin condoms," are made from animal tissue. Lambskin condoms don't protect you from HIV and other STIs. Make sure the package says "latex condom." The condom is the only form of birth control that men can use to prevent pregnancy. The condom and the female condom are the only birth control methods that protect against STIs.

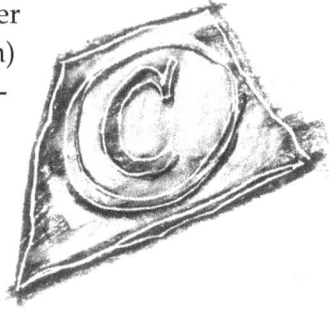

Effectiveness: Of 100 women whose partners use condoms when they have sex, about 15 will become pregnant during the first year of typical use. Typical use rates take into account that most people won't use condoms correctly every time. Using condoms correctly includes putting one on before you start rubbing up against each other naked (because semen can leak out of the penis before a man cums). It also means being careful about how you put the condom on and take it off. Being careful is worth it: Only 2 in every 100 women will become pregnant if condoms are used perfectly.

Because condoms help protect against HIV and other infections, anyone who is having vaginal (penis in vagina) or anal (penis in anus) sex should use them. To protect against STIs, you should also use a condom during oral (penis in mouth) sex.

Because it can break or slip off if not used correctly, the condom is more effective as birth control when used with spermicide, which is a sperm-killing foam, film, cream, insert, or jelly. Some condoms come with spermicide already inside them; the label will say "spermicidal lubricant."

Pros: Condoms help prevent the spread of HIV and other STIs. They are inexpensive and easy to get. You can buy them at any drugstore without a prescription, and many clinics and some high schools make them available for free. Since condoms are small and lightweight, it's easy to carry them with you at all times. They make it possible for men to take responsibility for birth control. They may also help a man stay erect longer.

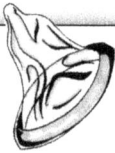

Condom Tips

- If a condom fails, both partners should wash their genitals with soap and water and urinate. Quickly applying a spermicide may also help.
- Even if you do it right, the condom can break. To avoid rips, use a water-based lubricant or a pre-lubricated condom. Do not use oil-based lubricants like cooking oil, baby oil, lotion, or petroleum jelly—they'll cause the condom to break.
- Extra-strength condoms are recommended for anal sex.
- Many condom packages print information about how to use a condom on the inside of the box. Open the package without too much ripping so you can carefully read the instructions and warnings.
- Condoms should be stored in a cool, dry place (not in wallets.) Heat, light, pressure, and air pollution can damage them.

Cons: You have to use one every time you have intercourse. Putting the condom on may feel awkward or uncomfortable at first since it must be used right at the time of intercourse. It may also dull sensation for either partner. It may tear or come off during intercourse, especially if it's not put on correctly (see directions on pages 96 and 97).

Possible Side Effects: There are none, except for people who are allergic to latex. (They can use plastic condoms, which are just as effective as latex.)

Cost: Condoms cost $7–13 per dozen at drugstores and supermarkets. Many clinics give them out for free.

THE FEMALE CONDOM

Description: A plastic baggie-like pouch that has flexible rings on each end. One ring is inserted deep into the vagina and the other ring stays open outside the vagina. The rings help to hold the condom in place.

The female condom collects semen before, during, and after ejaculation, keeping sperm from entering the vagina and protecting against pregnancy and STIs. Female condoms should not be used at the same time as male condoms.

Effectiveness: With typical use, 21 out of every 100 women using female condoms will get pregnant in a year. With perfect use, 5 out of 100 will get pregnant. Spermicide increases effectiveness.

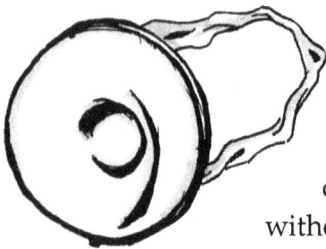

Pros: The female condom helps prevent many STIs (including HIV and AIDS), and can be used for both anal and vaginal sex. The female condom can be purchased at a drugstore without a prescription. It allows women to

Insertion of Female Condom

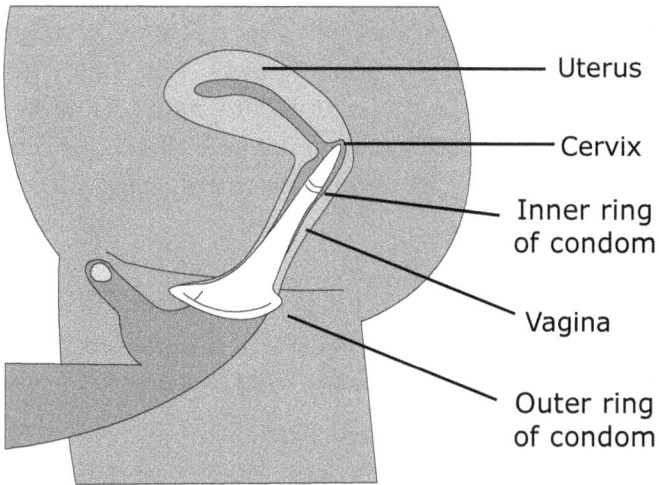

Uterus

Cervix

Inner ring of condom

Vagina

Outer ring of condom

For more detailed instructions, read the condom's package.

take responsibility for STI prevention without having to rely on their partners. And it can be used by people who are allergic to latex.

Cons: Female condoms can be tricky to use. They can only be used once. They are generally more expensive than male condoms.

Possible Side Effects: May cause irritation.

Price: You can pick up free female condoms at some clinics and other organizations. At a drugstore, a pack of three female condoms is about $17.

HORMONAL CONTRACEPTIVES

The pill, the patch, the ring, Depo-Provera, and Implanon are all forms of birth control that work by releasing hormones that prevent your body from producing eggs. When used correctly, they are very effective at preventing pregnancy. However, **none of these methods protect against HIV and other STIs.** To protect yourself from infection, you must also use a condom.

THE PILL

Description: A monthly series of pills—you take one birth control tablet a day. Basically, the pill has hormones that prevent pregnancy by stopping the release of eggs from your ovaries.

Effectiveness: With typical use, 8 women out of 100 will get pregnant while taking the pill. With perfect use (taking it every day at the same time), fewer than 1 out of 100 women will become pregnant. However, it may take a week or two for the pill to become effective.

Pros: The pill is good for women who are disciplined (because you have to remember to take it at the same time every day—missing a pill can lead to pregnancy). Women who use the pill have more regular periods, less menstrual flow, less cramping, less iron deficiency and anemia, less pelvic inflammatory disease (PID), and less premenstrual tension than women who don't take it. Also, it can reduce acne.

Cons: The pill doesn't protect against HIV or other STIs. You need a doctor's prescription to get the pill. You must take it every day at the same time, even when you aren't planning to have sex. Women who take it

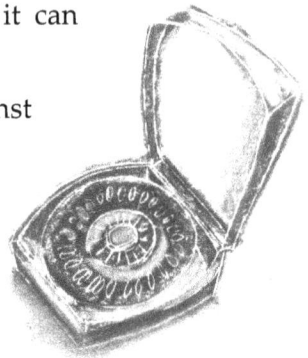

may be at slightly greater risk for some medical conditions like blood clots, heart attack, and stroke—ask your doctor about this. Smoking increases your risk for some of these conditions, so doctors recommend that you do not smoke when you are on the pill.

Possible Side Effects: Many women don't have any side effects, and for those who do, most side effects go away after two or three months. The pill can cause nausea, vomiting, headaches, mood changes, weight gain or loss, breast tenderness, or bleeding between periods.

Price: The pill costs anywhere from $15–50 a month, depending on what kind you take, whether or not it's covered by your insurance, and whether you buy it at a drugstore or a clinic. (Clinics are usually cheaper and sometimes offer a reduced rate based on income.) You must have a prescription.

There are several other, less popular kinds of hormonal contraceptive methods, including the patch, the ring, Depo-Provera, and Implanon. Like the pill, none of these methods prevent sexually transmitted infections, but they are highly effective in preventing pregnancy. All the hormonal contraceptives require a prescription. A brief overview of each:

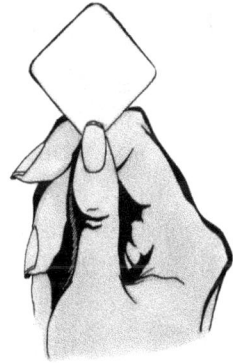

THE PATCH

The patch is a thin piece of plastic that is worn on the buttocks, stomach, upper arm, or upper torso (but never on the breasts). Use one patch per week for three weeks in a row. On the fourth week, you don't wear a patch and you get your period. Side effects are similar to the pill. It's about $15–50 per month.

THE RING

The ring is a soft and flexible plastic ring that's inserted into the vagina. Only one ring is needed for three weeks of use, though you must remember to remove it exactly 21 days after you put it in, and replace it one week after that. Inserting the ring may be awkward at first. Side effects may include mood swings, headache, nausea, vaginal discharge, breast tenderness, weight gain or loss, bleeding between periods, and vaginal irritation. It is also about $15–50 a month.

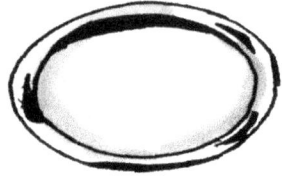

With typical use 8 women out of 100 will get pregnant while using the ring or the patch. With perfect use, fewer than 1 out of 100 women will become pregnant.

DEPO-PROVERA

Depo-Provera is a shot that you get injected into your body every 11–13 weeks with a needle. That means, you only have to worry about birth control four times a year. However, if you don't like it and want to stop using it, you'll have to suffer through any side effects you've been experiencing for up to three months while waiting for your last injection to wear off. Irregular periods are common. Less common side effects may include increased appetite and weight gain, headache, sore breasts, nausea, nervousness, dizziness, depression, skin rashes or spotty darkening of the skin, hair loss, increased hair on face or body, and increased or decreased sex drive.

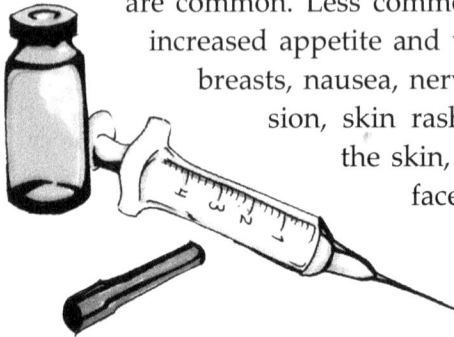

The initial doctor's visit to get Depo-Provera can be $35–250 and injections are $35–75 four times a year. You may have to pay exam fees between $20–40 during each visit, as well. You should not use it continuously for more than two years.

IMPLANON

Another highly effective hormonal birth control method is **Implanon**, or implantable contraception. Implanon is a small, matchstick-sized flexible plastic tube containing hormones that doctors insert just under the skin of the upper arm. It protects against pregnancy for up to three years. However, it's expensive. The cost of the exam, Implanon, and insertion ranges from $400–800. Removal costs around $100. Medicaid and private health insurance may cover it. Possible side effects are similar to the pill, plus irritation, infection, and possible scarring where the tubes are inserted.

Both Depo-Provera and Implanon are convenient and highly effective—fewer than 1 out of 100 women who use them correctly will get pregnant.

BARRIER METHOD CONTRACEPTIVES

Like condoms, the diaphragm and cervical cap help prevent pregnancy by blocking sperm from entering the uterus. However, **neither of these methods protect against HIV and other STIs**. To protect yourself from infection, you must also use a condom.

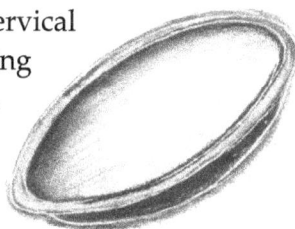

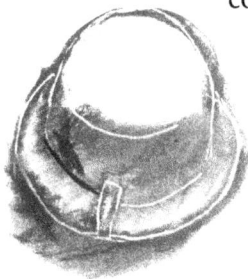

The **diaphragm** is a soft silicone or latex cup that you fill with spermicide and insert into the vagina up to six hours before sex. A **cervical cap** is similar to a diaphragm, but smaller, and can be inserted up to 40

hours before sex. You must see a doctor and get fitted to get one. There are almost no side effects or health risks for either of these methods, but they are less effective than hormonal birth control: Out of 100 women who use them, 14–16 will become pregnant during the first year of typical use.

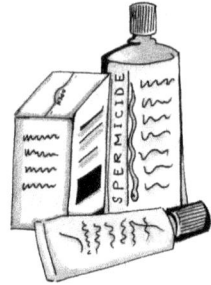

Both barrier methods must be used with spermicide, a sperm-killing chemical that can be bought at drugstores. Spermicides come in many forms, including film, inserts, foam, cream, and jelly, and cost about $8-18 per tube. A tube will last a while.

Rasheeda was 20 and Kymberly was 17 when they wrote this story. Rasheeda went on to earn a degree in Economics from the University of Virginia; Kymberly went to the State University of New York at Purchase.

Resources

Planned Parenthood offers confidential services to teens regardless of age or income, including GYN exams, all kinds of contraceptives, family planning counseling, emergency birth control, pregnancy testing, prenatal care, abortions, and STI and HIV testing. For the Planned Parenthood nearest you, call 1-800-230-PLAN or check www.plannedparenthood.org.

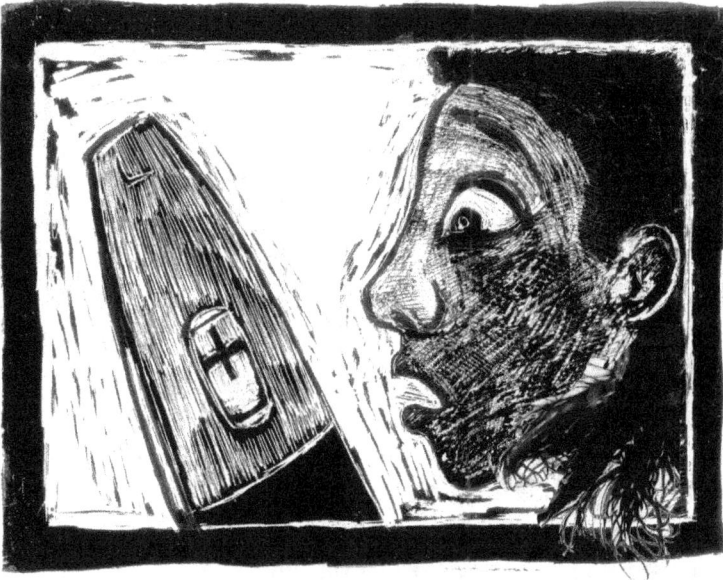

Pregnant? Explore Your Options

Finding out that you are pregnant can be emotional and confusing. Whether the pregnancy was planned or not, it's common to feel a range of emotions, such as fear, anger, happiness, guilt, confusion, excitement, and sadness. Once you find out you're pregnant, you have some big decisions to make. The three options you have are:

- Continue the pregnancy and raise the child
- Continue the pregnancy and put the child up for adoption
- Discontinue the pregnancy (have an abortion)

It's important to weigh all of your options, examine your values about each option, and talk to people you trust. Even if you got pregnant on purpose, you still have a chance to change your mind about raising the child, or you may be questioning your options. Whatever you decide, we hope this information will help you find the support you need.

Becoming a Parent

Many teens end up having kids before they're ready. I was 14 when I gave birth to my daughter, and I had to change a lot. I had to learn to be patient and responsible.

If you're having sex without using protection, or if you're thinking about having a baby, ask yourself the questions I wish I'd asked myself: Am I working and living in my own apartment? Am I in love with my child's father? Have we been together for a long time? Does he have a job? Are we both well-educated? Are we independent?

Can we depend on each other? If not, are there other supportive adults in my life who will help me raise this child? If you can't answer "yes" to these questions, you might want to think twice about becoming a parent right now.

If you do decide to become a parent, take advice from someone in an older generation—someone who you think treats their children well. Try to pay attention to your child. And most of all, if you need help, ask for it.

—Shannel Walker

Adoption

Putting your child up for adoption is another alternative for pregnant teens who feel that they aren't ready to be parents.

There are three types of adoption. Open adoption is when the birth parents are allowed contact with the child, although the adoptive parents can control when visitation occurs. In semi-open adoption, birth parents are involved with the adoption agency in choosing a placement for the child, and birth parents are allowed to exchange letters and photos of themselves with the child. In closed adoption there is no contact between the child and birth parents.

If you are considering adoption, you should talk to a licensed adoption agency or adoption attorney to learn more about your options.

Abortion

All pregnant women, including teenagers, have the right to choose what is best for them, including ending the pregnancy with a surgical or medical abortion.

Abortion is not a substitute for birth control. To prevent another unintended pregnancy, it is important to choose an effective, ongoing birth control method and to begin using it immediately after an abortion.

To find an abortion provider in your area, call The National Abortion Federation Hotline, at 1-800-772-9100. You can also call Planned Parenthood at 1-800-230-PLAN.

Teens:
How to Get More Out of This Book

Self-help: The teens who wrote the stories in this book did so because they hope that telling their stories will help readers who are facing similar challenges. They want you to know that you are not alone, and that taking specific steps can help you manage or overcome very difficult situations. They've done their best to be clear about the actions that worked for them so you can see if they'll work for you.

Writing: You can also use the book to improve your writing skills. Each teen in this book wrote 5-10 drafts of his or her story before it was published. If you read the stories closely you'll see that the teens work to include a beginning, a middle, and an end, and good scenes, description, dialogue, and anecdotes (little stories). To improve your writing, take a look at how these writers construct their stories. Try some of their techniques in your own writing.

Resources on the Web

We will occasionally post Think About It questions on our website, www.youthcomm.org, to accompany stories in this and other Youth Communication books. We try out the questions with teens and post the ones they like best. Many teens report that writing answers to those questions in a journal is very helpful.

How to Use This Book in Staff Training

Staff say that reading these stories gives them greater insight into what teens are thinking and feeling, and new strategies for working with them. You can help the staff you work with by using these stories as case studies.

Select one story to read in the group, and ask staff to identify and discuss the main issue facing the teen. There may be disagreement about this, based on the background and experience of staff. That is fine. One point of the exercise is that teens have complex lives and needs. Adults can probably be more effective if they don't focus too narrowly and can see several dimensions of their clients.

Ask staff: What issues or feelings does the story provoke in them? What kind of help do they think the teen wants? What interventions are likely to be most promising? Least effective? Why? How would you build trust with the teen writer? How have other adults failed the teen, and how might that affect his or her willingness to accept help? What other resources would be helpful to this teen, such as peer support, a mentor, counseling, family therapy, etc?

Resources on the Web

From time to time we will post Think About It questions on our website, www.youthcomm.org, to accompany stories in this and other Youth Communication books. We try out the questions with teens and post the ones that they find most effective. We'll also post lessons for some of the stories. Adults can use the questions and lessons in workshops.

Teachers and Staff:
How to Use This Book in Groups

When working with teens individually or in groups, you can use these stories to help young people face difficult issues in a way that feels safe to them. That's because talking about the issues in the stories usually feels safer to teens than talking about those same issues in their own lives. Addressing issues through the stories allows for some personal distance; they hit close to home, but not too close. Talking about them opens up a safe place for reflection. As teens gain confidence talking about the issues in the stories, they usually become more comfortable talking about those issues in their own lives.

Below are general questions to guide your discussion. In most cases you can read a story and conduct a discussion in one 45-minute session. Teens are usually happy to read the stories aloud, with each teen reading a paragraph or two. (Allow teens to pass if they don't want to read.) It takes 10-15 minutes to read a story straight through. However, it is often more effective to let workshop participants make comments and discuss the story as you go along. The workshop leader may even want to annotate her copy of the story beforehand with key questions.

If teens read the story ahead of time or silently, it's good to break the ice with a few questions that get everyone on the same page: Who is the main character? How old is she? What happened to her? How did she respond? Another good starting question is: "What stood out for you in the story?" Go around the room and let each person briefly mention one thing.

Then move on to open-ended questions, which encourage participants to think more deeply about what the writers were feeling, the choices they faced, and the actions they took. There are no right or wrong answers to the open-ended questions.

Open-ended questions encourage participants to think about how the themes, emotions, and choices in the stories relate to their own lives. Here are some examples of open-ended questions that we have found to be effective. You can use variations of these questions with almost any story in this book.

—What main problem or challenge did the writer face?

—What choices did the teen have in trying to deal with the problem?

—Which way of dealing with the problem was most effective for the teen? Why?

—What strengths, skills, or resources did the teen use to address the challenge?

—If you were in the writer's shoes, what would you have done?

—What could adults have done better to help this young person?

—What have you learned by reading this story that you didn't know before?

—What, if anything, will you do differently after reading this story?

—What surprised you in this story?

—Do you have a different view of this issue, or see a different way of dealing with it, after reading this story? Why or why not?

Credits

The stories in this book originally appeared in the following
Youth Communication publications:

"Am I the Father?," by Anonymous, *New Youth Connections*, December 2003; "Growing Up Together," by Vanessa Sanchez, *Rise*, Summer 2007; "Three Tales of Teen Pregnancy," by Jezaida Rivera, *New Youth Connections*, November 2000; "Getting Some (Answers)," by Lenny Jones, *New Youth Connections*, March 1998; "Mom Wasn't Ready for Me," by Anonymous, *Represent*, July/August 2000; "The Morning After," by Anonymous, *New Youth Connections*, May/June 2002; "The Right Choice for Me—for Now," by Anonymous, *New Youth Connections*, September/October 1999; "A Family to Raise Her," by Jennifer Jeanne Olensky, *Represent*, May/June 2001; "Stressed About Sex," by G. Santos, *New Youth Connections*, May/June 2002; "There's More to Sex Than Sex," by Anonymous; *New Youth Connections*, September/October 1992; "A Difficult Decision," by Anonymous, *Represent*, May/June 2001; "Keeping My Baby," by Anonymous, *Represent*, July/August 2000; "A Choice I Couldn't Make," by DeAnna Lyles; "Why I Always Use a Condom," by Anonymous, *Strange Brew*, June 1992; "If You Believe These Lines, Check the Price of Pampers," by Frank Jones, *New Youth Connections*, September/October 1990; "Back in the Stirrups—Again," by Madeleine Gordillo, *Represent*, July/August 2005; "All About Birth Control, Right Here," by Rasheeda Raji and Kymberly Sheckleford, *New Youth Connections*, December 2003; "Pregnant? Explore Your Options," by Youth Communication.

About
Youth Communication

Youth Communication, founded in 1980, is a nonprofit youth development program located in New York City whose mission is to teach writing, journalism, and leadership skills. The teenagers we train become writers for our websites and books and for two print magazines: *New Youth Connections*, a general-interest youth magazine, and *Represent*, a magazine by and for young people in foster care.

Each year, up to 100 young people participate in Youth Communication's school-year and summer journalism workshops, where they work under the direction of full-time professional editors. Most are African-American, Latino, or Asian, and many are recent immigrants. The opportunity to reach their peers with accurate portrayals of their lives and important self-help information motivates the young writers to create powerful stories.

Our goal is to run a strong youth development program in which teens produce high quality stories that inform and inspire their peers. Doing so requires us to be sensitive to the complicated lives and emotions of the teen participants while also providing an intellectually rigorous experience. We achieve that goal in the writing/teaching/editing relationship, which is the core of our program.

Our teaching and editorial process begins with discussions

between adult editors and the teen staff. In those meetings, the teens and the editors work together to identify the most important issues in the teens' lives and to figure out how those issues can be turned into stories that will resonate with teen readers.

Once story topics are chosen, students begin the process of crafting their stories. For a personal story, that means revisiting events in one's past to understand their significance for the future. For a commentary, it means developing a logical and persuasive point of view. For a reported story, it means gathering information through research and interviews. Students look inward and outward as they try to make sense of their experiences and the world around them and find the points of intersection between personal and social concerns. That process can take a few weeks or a few months. Stories frequently go through ten or more drafts as students work under the guidance of their editors, the way any professional writer does.

Many of the students who walk through our doors have uneven skills, as a result of poor education, living under extremely stressful conditions, or coming from homes where English is a second language. Yet, to complete their stories, students must successfully perform a wide range of activities, including writing and rewriting, reading, discussion, reflection, research, interviewing, and typing. They must work as members of a team and they must accept individual responsibility. They learn to provide constructive criticism, and to accept it. They engage in explorations of truthfulness, fairness, and accuracy. They meet deadlines. They must develop the audacity to believe that they have something important to say and the humility to recognize that saying it well is not a process of instant gratification. Rather, it usually requires a long, hard struggle through many discussions and much rewriting.

It would be impossible to teach these skills and dispositions as separate, disconnected topics, like grammar, ethics, or assertiveness. However, we find that students make rapid progress when they are learning skills in the context of an inquiry that is personally significant to them and that will benefit their peers.

When teens publish their stories—in *New Youth Connections* and *Represent*, on the Web, and in other publications—they reach tens of thousands of teen and adult readers. Teachers, counselors, social workers, and other adults circulate the stories to young people in their classes and out-of-school youth programs. Adults tell us that teens in their programs—including many who are ordinarily resistant to reading—clamor for the stories. Teen readers report that the stories give them information they can't get anywhere else, and inspire them to reflect on their lives and open lines of communication with adults.

Writers usually participate in our program for one semester, though some stay much longer. Years later, many of them report that working here was a turning point in their lives—that it helped them acquire the confidence and skills that they needed for success in college and careers. Scores of our graduates have overcome tremendous obstacles to become journalists, writers, and novelists. They include National Book Award finalist and MacArthur Fellowship winner Edwidge Danticat, novelist Ernesto Quiñonez, writer Veronica Chambers, and *New York Times* reporter Rachel Swarns. Hundreds more are working in law, business, and other careers. Many are teachers, principals, and youth workers, and several have started nonprofit youth programs themselves and work as mentors—helping another generation of young people develop their skills and find their voices.

Youth Communication is a nonprofit educational corporation. Contributions are gratefully accepted and are tax deductible to the fullest extent of the law.

To make a contribution, or for information about our publications and programs, including our catalog of over 100 books and curricula for hard-to-reach teens, see www.youthcomm.org.

About the Editors

Maria Luisa Tucker is the associate editor of *New Youth Connections*, Youth Communication's magazine by and for New York City teens. Before coming to Youth Communication, she worked as a reporter for *Village Voice*. She has also written for several other publications, including *AlterNet.org*, an online magazine, and the *Santa Fe Reporter*, a weekly newspaper where her work garnered several awards for investigative and media reporting. She holds a bachelor's degree in journalism from Texas State University and a master's in American Studies from Columbia University.

Keith Hefner co-founded Youth Communication in 1980 and has directed it ever since. He is the recipient of the Luther P. Jackson Education Award from the New York Association of Black Journalists and a MacArthur Fellowship. He was also a Revson Fellow at Columbia University.

Laura Longhine is the editorial director at Youth Communication. She edited *Represent*, Youth Communication's magazine by and for youth in foster care, for three years, and has written for a variety of publications. She has a BA in English from Tufts University and an MS in Journalism from Columbia University.

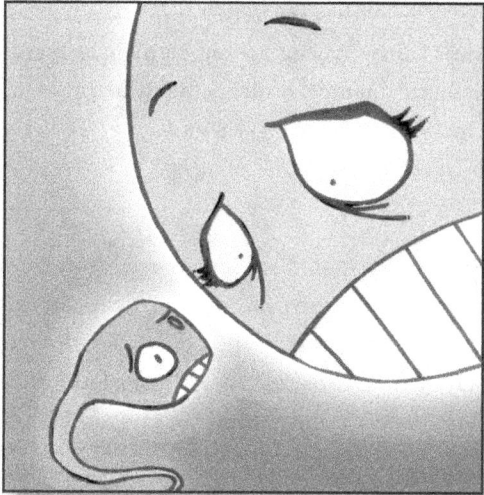

More Helpful Books
From Youth Communication

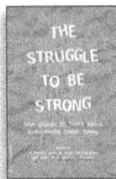

The Struggle to Be Strong: True Stories by Teens About Overcoming Tough Times. Foreword by Veronica Chambers. Help young people identify and build on their own strengths with 30 personal stories about resiliency. (Free Spirit)

Starting With "I": Personal Stories by Teenagers. "Who am I and who do I want to become?" Thirty-five stories examine this question through the lens of race, ethnicity, gender, sexuality, family, and more. Increase this book's value with the free Teacher's Guide, available from youthcomm.org. (Youth Communication)

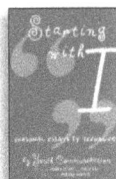

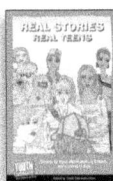

Real Stories, Real Teens. Inspire teens to read and recognize their strengths with this collection of 26 true stories by teens. The young writers describe how they overcame significant challenges and stayed true to themselves. Also includes the first chapters from three novels in the Bluford Series. (Youth Communication)

Out With It: Gay and Straight Teens Write About Homosexuality. Break stereotypes and provide support with this unflinching look at gay life from a teen's perspective. With a focus on urban youth, this book also includes several heterosexual teens' transformative experiences with gay peers. (Youth Communication)

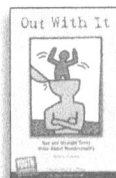

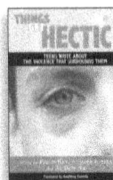

Things Get Hectic: Teens Write About the Violence That Surrounds Them. Violence is commonplace in many teens' lives, be it bullying, gangs, dating, or family relationships. Hear the experiences of victims, perpetrators, and witnesses through more than 50 real-world stories. (Youth Communication)

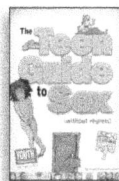

The Teen Guide to Sex (without regrets). Help teens understand that sex isn't something that just happens to them—they have choices. These teen writers answer common questions, and describe how becoming sexually active has changed their lives, for better or worse. (Youth Communication)

Am I Ready: Girls Write About Sex. Help teen girls make thoughtful choices about sex and relationships by using these stories as a jumping-off point for discussion. (Youth Communication)

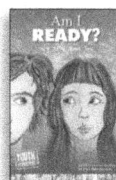

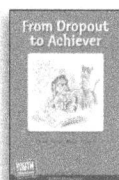

From Dropout to Achiever: Teens Write About School. Help teens overcome the challenges of graduating, which may involve overcoming family problems, bouncing back from a bad semester, or even dropping out for a time. These teens show how they achieve academic success. (Youth Communication)

Why I'm Still a Virgin: Teens Write About Saying No to Sex (Or Wishing They Had). Teens share why they have chosen to abstain from sex, often in the face of extreme peer pressure. They have a variety of reasons—fear, religion, morals, family values, or just a personal sense that they're not ready. (Youth Communication)

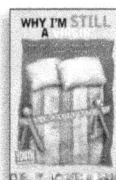

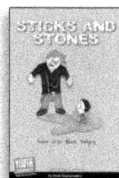

Sticks and Stones: Teens Write About Bullying. Shed light on bullying, as told from the perspectives of the bully, the victim, and the witness. These stories show why bullying occurs, the harm it causes, and how it might be prevented. (Youth Communication)

Through Thick and Thin: Teens Write About Obesity, Eating Disorders, and Self Image. Help teens who struggle with obesity, eating disorders, and body image issues. These stories show the pressures teens face when they are confronted by unrealistic standards for physical appearance, and how emotions can affect the way we eat. (Youth Communication)

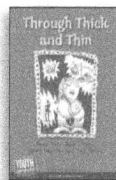

To order these and other books, go to:
www.youthcomm.org
or call 212-279-0708 x115

www.ingramcontent.com/pod-product-compliance
Lightning Source LLC
Chambersburg PA
CBHW052038270326
41931CB00012B/2542